Dr. Earl Mindell's
GOJI
The Asian Health Secret
THIRD EDITION

Earl Mindell, R.Ph., M.H., Ph.D.

Basic Health
PUBLICATIONS, INC.

The information contained in this book is based upon the research and personal and professional experiences of the authors. It is not intended as a substitute for consulting with your physician or other healthcare provider. Any attempt to diagnose and treat an illness should be done under the direction of a healthcare professional.

The publisher does not advocate the use of any particular healthcare protocol but believes the information in this book should be available to the public. The publisher and authors are not responsible for any adverse effects or consequences resulting from the use of the suggestions, preparations, or procedures discussed in this book. Should the reader have any questions concerning the appropriateness of any procedures or preparation mentioned, the authors and the publisher strongly suggest consulting a professional healthcare advisor.

Basic Health Publications, Inc.
28812 Top of the World Drive
Laguna Beach, CA 92651
949-715-7327 • www.basichealthpub.com

Library of Congress Cataloging-in-Publication Data
Mindell, Earl.
    Goji : the Asian health secret / Earl Mindell, R.Ph., M.H., Ph.D. —
Third edition.
        pages ; cm
    Includes bibliographical references and index.
    ISBN 978-1-59120-303-2
1. Fruit in human nutrition. 2. Berries—Health aspects. I. Title.
    QP144.F78M56   2013
    613.2—dc23
                                                          2012035473

Editor: Diana Drew
Typesetting/Book design: Gary A. Rosenberg
Cover design: Mike Stromberg

Printed in the United States of America

10   9   8   7   6   5   4   3   2   1

CONTENTS

ACKNOWLEDGMENTS

I would like to thank Dr. G. T. Wrench and Col. Reginald C. F. Schomberg, whose pioneering insights have led to the miraculous discoveries you will find within these pages.

Throughout the writing of this book, I was guided by the astute wisdom of the great Nobel laureate Dr. Albert Szent-Gyorgyi, who said,

> *"Discovery consists in seeing what everybody else*
> *has seen and thinking what nobody has thought."*

PREFACE

If you were given the choice, how long would you choose to live?

Eighty years? Ninety? One hundred-plus years? Perhaps even forever?

Unfortunately, we cannot live forever. Yet, in this age of modern medical miracles, it shouldn't be unreasonable to expect a long and relatively healthy life of at least 80 years, wouldn't you think?

The fact is the average citizen of Japan or Sweden has a significantly better chance of reaching that milestone than do those in most civilized Western countries. As the U.S. Census Bureau informs us, a mere 3.3 percent of the population will live to blow out the candles on our 80th birthday cake!

How Long Should We Expect to Live?

According to the National Center for Health Statistics, most of us can anticipate an average lifespan of just 78 years. That's not very reassuring. Even worse, a good number of those years may not be spent in prime health.

Chronic health conditions can have a serious impact on our ability to lead independent lives. The National Health Interview Survey found 20 percent of people between the ages of 55 and 64 to be limited in the ability to handle even basic personal care needs such as bathing or dressing. By ages 65 to 74, fully one-third of us may be impaired in our ability to walk, to remember, or to perform simple household chores. By age 75, nearly half of us will require some outside assistance.

% Affected by Chronic Health Conditions

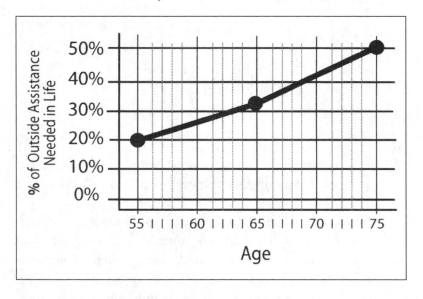

Winning the Longevity Game

Did you know that in some remote places in this world, a life expectancy of more than 100 years is not uncommon? More importantly, these people's lives are not merely long; they are also filled with abundant health and happiness.

Unlike most of us, they are virtually free from the ravages of high blood pressure, diabetes, heart disease, many types of cancer and the crippling pain of arthritis and degenerative disease.
Even in old age, their vision is sharp, they have boundless energy and strength, and their minds are clear.

Their vocabularies have no words for the debilitating conditions that have become all too familiar to our Western ears: *fibromyalgia, depression, anxiety, panic disorder, sexual dysfunction, chronic fatigue syndrome* . . . terms we wish we could purge from our vocabularies.

Who Are These People? Where Do They Live? What's Their Secret?

There are some small societies of extremely long-living people to be found in remote areas of the globe.

For example, a group of researchers from the Natural Science Institute have discovered a region on the West Elbow Plateau of the Yellow River in Inner Mongolia where people have lived to be more than 120 years old.

You say you haven't heard about them? That's probably because the Inner Mongolian West Elbow Plateau is not exactly a tourist destination. But the simple people of the West Elbow Plateau have something that we can't buy at any store or mega-mall: *longevity*.

Coffins for Storage Bins

The people of West Elbow are not the only ones to enjoy an extremely long life. Consider the residents of the tiny hamlet of Pinghan, nestled deep among a stand of limestone hills in a remote region of southwestern China. In Pinghan, locals honor an old tradition of buying a coffin at the age of 61. The coffins are kept in or around the home, and most villagers get many decades of use out of them, employing them as storage bins or hampers before finally pressing them into service as eternal resting places. That's because the people of Pinghan and the surrounding county are exceptionally long-lived. The county has more than 74 centenarians and 237 residents who have reached their 90s. That's one of the highest *per capita* concentrations of old-timers in the world, according to Chen Jinchao, a surgeon who, for the past 10 years, has run the Guangxi Bama Long Life Research Institute.

Extreme longevity and health are not exclusive to just these two small tribal villages. There are actually a small handful of long-lived cultures scattered across the mountains of Asia. Although the inhabitants of each of these pockets of longevity might not know of the existence of the others, they all share some important common traits:

- They live in isolated and sometimes inaccessible places, away from the more harmful influences of modern Western civilization. In other words, long-lived cultures don't know what it means to eat processed or "fast foods."

- Their diet contains fresh fruits, vegetables and whole grains, and it is low in animal fats.

- Most important, many of the world's longest living people consume regular daily helpings of a tiny red fruit that just happens to be the world's most powerful anti-aging food: the *goji berry*.

YOU'VE NEVER HEARD OF A GOJI BERRY?

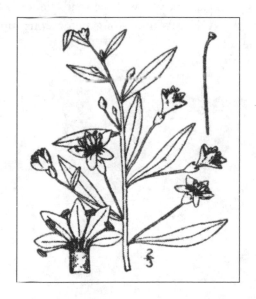

You're not alone, but that's about to change. This little red berry is about to open your eyes. By the time you finish this book, you will want to join in celebration with the people of Central Asia who love and cherish these berries so much that they *devote two weeks every year to festivals* in their honor (similar to a Bavarian Oktoberfest, but a lot healthier . . . and just as happy!).

There is good reason for the locals to honor the goji berry. After thousands of years of use, those who use the berry are still awed by its unmatched healing and protective powers. They celebrate as a continuing acknowledgement of just how much their very lives depend upon it. No medicinal plant in all of Asian medicine can approach goji for its incredible diversity of legendary benefits.

And as far back as the 1830s, Europe was also catching onto the amazing benefits of this tiny red fruit. It was first described by J. Harvey von Bloom in *Folk Lore, Old Customs and Superstitions in Shakespeare Land, London*. In fact, the fruit was tied as beads around the necks of teething children to help ease their pain.

It's a medical shame that so many centuries have passed without the benefits of this amazing little berry being shared with the world. But as you read on, you will see that science is finally confirming what the Ancients knew long before our modern drugs came onto the scene.

CHAPTER 1

MODERN RESEARCH CONFIRMS ANCIENT WISDOM

Many of the traditional health-giving properties of the goji berry are being confirmed in modern scientific studies, and this has led to the discovery of even more far-reaching benefits. These health-giving properties are listed here, and discussed in detail in later chapters.

Top 34 Health Benefits of Goji

1. Extends your life, protecting your body from premature aging through its powerful antioxidant action

2. Increases your energy and strength, especially when fighting disease

3. Makes you look and feel younger. Goji stimulates the secretion of hGH (human growth hormone), the "youth hormone."

4. Lowers your blood pressure

5. Prevents cancer

6. Maintains healthy cholesterol levels

7. Balances blood sugar and manages diabetes

8. Enhances libido and sexual function

9. Helps you lose weight

10. Relieves headaches and dizziness

11. Helps you get better sleep

12. Improves your vision

13. Strengthens your heart

14. Inhibits lipid peroxidation. Accumulation of sticky lipid per-oxides in the blood can lead to cardiovascular disease, heart attack, atherosclerosis and stroke. Goji increases levels of an important blood enzyme that inhibits their formation.

15. Aids in disease resistance

16. Improves immune response by balancing the activity of all classes of immune cells, including T-cells, cytotoxic T-cells, NK cells, lysozyme, tumor necrosis factor-alpha and the immunoglobulins IgG and IgA

17. Manages and fights cancer, including regressions of malignant melanoma, renal cell carcinoma, colorectal carcinoma, lung cancer, nasopharyngeal carcinoma and malignant hydrothorax

18. Protects your precious DNA, the most important chemical in your body, ensuring that—as they need replacement—your 10 trillion cells are faithfully reproduced as healthy, exact duplicates, and restoring and repairing damaged DNA

19. Inhibits tumor growth

20. Reduces the toxic effects of chemotherapy and radiation

21. Builds strong blood, enhancing production of red blood cells, white blood cells and platelets

22. Helps chronic dry cough

23. Fights inflammation and arthritis by restoring the balance of the important anti-inflammatory SOD enzyme

24. Improves your lymphocyte count. A lymphocyte is any of a group of white blood cells important to the adaptive part of the body's immune system. Goji increases lymphocyte count.

25. Treats menopausal symptoms

26. Prevents morning sickness in the first trimester of pregnancy

27. Improves fertility

28. Strengthens your muscles and bones

29. Supports kidney health

30. Improves your memory

31. Supports healthy liver function

32. Alleviates anxiety and stress

33. Promotes cheerfulness and brighten your spirit, explaining why goji is called the "happy berry." In fact, it has been noted that the only known side effect of goji is that continued consumption may make it impossible for you to stop smiling!

34. Improves digestion

CHAPTER 2

IN SEARCH OF
THE TRUE GOJI

When scientific studies were first initiated to confirm the traditionally observed benefits of goji berries, they did not yield uniformly positive results. It could have been foreseen that these studies would arrive at inconsistent conclusions, as they were performed using the whole dried berries.

There can be tremendous variation in the quality of dried fruits, depending upon how they were harvested, dehydrated and stored, and also depending upon the quality of the fresh berries from which they were made. While goji berries grow in a lot of places, their quality can vary enormously.

The same is true in the growing of wine grapes. How is it that the Chardonnay grapes of one vineyard will yield a spectacular vintage, while the same grapes in a neighboring field will produce wines that are merely ordinary? A few minutes more of daily sunshine or a little better drainage in one field or the other can make all the difference between a $100 bottle of Dom Perignon and a $10 bottle of "bargain bubbly."

A Gaggle of Goji Berries

Just as there are many varieties of grapes, there are also many varieties of goji berries to be found growing in different parts of the world. It has been claimed that there are 41 species in Tibet alone. Each has its own distinctive appearance, color and taste, and each may differ from others in its medicinal power. Some of them are unrelated, coming from different botanical families.

Variants of the goji vine have been found in the fjords of Norway and the Arizona desert, in Inner Mongolia and in Outer Patagonia.

Could this be any more confusing? Researchers seeking to unlock the secrets of the goji berry were perplexed. They knew that only consistently excellent berries could yield consistently excellent clinical results, but which of the dozens of varieties were the best?

Of all the species known as goji, researchers decided to concentrate their efforts only on those that came from the botanical family known as *Solanaceae*. They further narrowed their choices to include only the desert-thorns of the genus *Lycium* (lye-SEE-um).

Their choices were made from a historical perspective, based on descriptions of goji in ancient medical texts. In fact, goji was declared to be a superior herb as early as the first century A.D., when it was extolled in the *Divine Farmer's Handbook of Natural Medicine (Shen Nong Ben Cao)*, perhaps the most important text in the history of Chinese medicine.

Interestingly, Tao Hong Jing (456–536 A.D.), a Taoist master, wrote a treatise called *Commentary on the Divine Farmer's Handbook of Natural Medicine*. Tao Hong Jing tells us that "*Lycium* tonifies *jing* (vital energy) and *qi* (breath) and strengthens the *yin tao* (capacity for physical exercise) within a human."

Those early endorsements were so powerful that even to this day, people not only in China but all throughout Asia use the fruit of the *Lycium* goji plant as a potent anti-aging herb. Many who eat the berry or drink its juice every day will tell you of its history and legend. Most often, they will relate the tale of the most famous goji user of all time, Master Li Qing Yuen.

CHAPTER 3

LI QING YUEN:
A SHORT STORY ABOUT
A VERY LONG LIFE

There is an incredible Chinese longevity story in which *Lycium* plays a starring role, and it's cited as one of the primary reasons for the preeminence of goji in Chinese medicine, which continues to the present day.

The legend centers around a gentleman named Li Qing Yuen, who is said to have lived to be 252 years old. In case you think that this is one of those Chinese fables that supposedly happened long before the invention of paper, ink and witnesses, such is not the case. Li Qing Yuen was born in relatively modern times by Chinese standards, in the year 1678, and his incredible lifespan has been documented and verified by modern scholars.

We know that Li Qing Yuen was born in the mountainous southwest of China, a remote and harsh area not well suited for a boy of his adventurous and wandering nature. When three traveling herbalists chanced to visit his village, young Li, barely 11 years old, seized upon the opportunity and begged the three men to allow him to follow them on their journeys. His passion and inquisitive nature soon won over the older men, and they accepted him as an apprentice.

Together the boy and his three teachers traveled throughout China, Tibet, and Southeast Asia. Li Qing Yuen became an expert in the herbal traditions of all these various regions.

Perhaps no one tells the legend of Li Qing Yuen better than the noted master Chinese herbalist Ron Teeguarden in *The Ancient Wisdom of the Chinese Tonic Herbs*, who writes:

> *"Because of his herbal expertise, Master Li was well known for his amazing vigor and excellent health. Then one day, when he was around 50 years old, while out on a hike, he met a very old man who, in spite of his venerable old age, could out-walk Li Qing Yuen. This impressed Master Li very much because he believed that brisk walking was both a way to health and longevity and a sign of inner health. Li Qing Yuen inquired as to the old sage's secret. He was told that if he consumed a 'soup' of Lycium every day, he would soon attain a new standard of health. Li Qing Yuen did just that and continued to consume the soup daily.*
>
> *"Naturally, he was greatly revered by all those who knew him and he had many disciples who followed him. Even at a very old age, his sight was keen and his legs were strong, and he continued to take his daily vigorous walks. One day, he was on a journey through treacherous mountains. In the mountains he met a Taoist hermit who claimed to be five hundred years old. Humbled by the great illumination of the old Taoist, Li Qing Yuen begged the sage to tell him his secrets. The old Taoist, recognizing the sincerity of Li, taught him the secrets of Taoist Yoga . . .*
>
> *"He continued to consume his Lycium soup daily. It is said that Master Li also changed his diet so as to consume little meat or root vegetables and limited his consumption of grain. Instead, he lived mainly on steamed aboveground vegetables and herbs. He lived to be 252 years old, dying in 1930, reportedly after a banquet presented in his honor by a government official."*

Whatever the cause of death, Li Qing Yuen had lived an amazingly long life. He had married 14 times, and had lived to see 11 generations of descendants, who numbered nearly 200!

The story of Li Qing Yuen is a powerful testimony to the remarkable berry that the Chinese call goji (spelled *gouqi*, or sometimes seen as *gouqizi*), and which is also known by its Latin name of *Lycium*.

Why Latin?

Latin is the universal language that botanists around the world use to classify and categorize plants. *Lycium* is what is known as the *genus* name. A genus is a group of plants that are closely related and share similar characteristics. For example, all trees in the Pine genus (*Pinus*) have long, narrow needles bound in bundles and hard, woody cones with thick, tough scales. Within the Pine genus you'll find different varieties such as the Ponderosa pine, White pine and Scotch pine. These individual types are called *species*.

The same holds true for *Lycium*. Within the family there are dozens of different species, but there are only two primary types of *Lycium* goji berries that are used medicinally.

CHAPTER 4

THE TWO PRINCIPAL
GOJI TYPES

The first type of goji is called *Lycium chinense*, which grows mainly in Hebei province in China. The berries are small, orange to light red in color, and have many seeds. They are too sour to eat as is, so they are added to foods. *Lycium chinense* is sometimes referred to as Chinese wolfberry, matrimony vine, or Chinese boxthorn.

The second, and more important type of true goji berry—the one that is said to have the best effect—is known as *Lycium barbarum*.

It grows in various regions of Asia such as Tibet and Inner Mongolia, but nowhere is the *Lycium barbarum* goji berry revered more than in Ningxia, situated along the Yellow River between the Yinchuan plain, the Helan mountains and the Maowusu desert in the western part of China.

Ningxia: Goji Capital of the World?

Ningxia has an unusually alkaline soil (pH 8.2–8.6), and an extreme temperature range of from 102°F to –16°F (38.5°C to –27°C). That might not sound comfortable to you, but it's like heaven to a goji vine, and it brings out the best in them.

Ningxia goji berries are a real treat. The fruits are large and plump, with a beautiful deep red color, few seeds and an exquisitely sweet taste and juicy texture.

The people of Ningxia are simply crazy about their goji berries, which have always grown wild on the hillsides, and which they have been cultivating in rows for more than 500 years.

In Ningxia, goji legends based on history and tradition abound. One story tells of the people of the small village of Nanqiu, who were exceedingly fond of goji. The residents of Nanqiu bore testament to the longevity attributes of goji, as, at one time, there were more than 10 villagers who had reached one hundred years of age! The county magistrate reported the matter to the emperor, who bestowed upon Nanqiu the title of "Long Life Village."

In Ningxia, poems have been written to honor goji. These poems reflect the known secrets and serious nature with which ancient people regarded goji.

There's actually a rather well-known poem that was written by the noted Tang Dynasty poet Liu Yuxi (772–842 A.D.). At a famous Buddhist temple, a well had been dug beside a wall that was covered with goji vines. Over the years, countless berries had fallen into the well. Those who prayed there had ruddy complexions, and even at the age of 80 they had no white hair and had not lost any teeth, simply because they would drink the water from the well. From this legend, Liu Yuxi crafted his poem:

The Goji Well

a cool well beside the monk's house
a clear spring feeds the well and the water has great powers
emerald green leaves grow on the wall
the deep red berries shine like copper
the flourishing branch like a walking stick
the old root in a dog's shape signals good fortune
the goji nourishes body and spirit
drink of the well and enjoy a long life

Makes you want to pluck some berries from a Ningxia goji vine, doesn't it? Well, before you do, you should know that today, many believe that the best Ningxia-type berries don't even come from

Ningxia. Instead, it is argued that the best Ningxia goji berries come from the very western end of China, in the region known as Xinjiang.

So Much for "The Goji Capital of the World"

The name Xinjiang may look like Ningxia spelled sideways, but it is a separate autonomous region that lies at the foot of the Tianshan, or "Heavenly Mountains"—a range that nearly equals the Himalayan mountain peaks. The pure snow runoff is the only water used to grow the goji berries in this region. They are said to be of a quality that is simply unattainable by berries grown anywhere else on earth.

The residents of Ningxia respectfully disagree, as do those of the other regions in the Chinese *goji belt:* Hebei, Gansu, Qinghai and Shanxi. They all believe that their berries are simply the best, and they can take it very personally if you insist otherwise.

It's hard to settle such a dispute, especially when civic pride is concerned. This "battle of the berries" is not new in China. If you can imagine, it was a hot debate even in the year 1590, when herbalist Li Shizhen wrote his *Book of Medicinal Herbs* (Ben Cao Gang Mu). Li tells us that in the most ancient times, the best goji berries came from Changshan. That all changed in the Tang Dynasty (618–907 A.D.), which saw a goji power shift to Shandong and Hebei. At the time Li Shizhen wrote his book, during the Ming Dynasty (1368–1644 A.D.), Shanxi and Gansu were considered to be the "in" places for great goji berries.

Goji supremacy is also claimed by the Tibetans, as well as by the Inner Mongolians, and let's not forget to mention the Koreans, who call their berry *kugicha*, and the Japanese, who know it as *kukoshi*.

CHAPTER 5

GOJI GOES UNDER
THE MICROSCOPE

For the scientists trying to unlock the secrets of the goji berry, it quickly became apparent that there was probably no one "best" growing region. Therefore, they decided to do what scientists do. They determined that they would pull the goji berry apart in the laboratory. They dissected it to find out what makes it tick.

The goji researchers began with some simple vitamin, mineral and nutrient analysis, expecting to find results similar to other fruits. They were totally unprepared for what they found. This tiny fruit revealed itself to be quite possibly the most nutritionally dense food on earth!

Goji Facts:

- Contains 19 amino acids—the building blocks of protein— including all eight that are essential for life.

- Contains 21 trace minerals, including germanium, an anti-cancer trace mineral rarely found in foods.

- Contains more protein than whole wheat (13 percent).

- Contains a complete spectrum of antioxidant *carotenoids*, including *beta-carotene* (a better source than even carrots!) and *zeaxanthin* (protects the eyes). Goji berries are the richest source of carotenoids of all known foods.

- Contains vitamin C at higher levels than even those found in oranges.

- Contains B-complex vitamins, necessary for converting food into energy.

- Contains vitamin E (very rarely found in fruits, only in grains and seeds).

- Contains beta-sitosterol, an anti-inflammatory agent. Beta-sitosterol also lowers cholesterol and has been used to treat sexual impotence and prostate enlargement.

- Contains essential fatty acids, which are required for the body's production of hormones and for the smooth functioning of the brain and nervous system.

- Contains cyperone, a sesquiterpene that benefits the heart and blood pressure, alleviates menstrual discomfort, and has been used in the treatment of cervical cancer.

- Contains solavetivone, a powerful anti-fungal and anti-bacterial compound.

- Contains physalin, a natural compound that is active against all major types of leukemia. It has been shown to increase splenic natural killer cell activity in normal and tumor-bearing mice, with broad-spectrum anticancer effect. It has also been used as a treatment for hepatitis B.

- Contains betaine, which is used by the liver to produce choline, a compound that calms nervousness, enhances memory, promotes muscle growth, and protects against fatty liver disease. Betaine also provides methyl groups in the body's energy reactions and can help reduce levels of homocysteine, a prime risk factor in heart disease. It also protects DNA.

Goji Plays "Hard to Get"

Even with its extensive and diverse nutrient profile revealed, the goji still seemed to be holding on to some secrets. There appeared to be many therapeutic effects that simply could not be explained.

This was not a big surprise. With medicinal herbs, activity is hardly ever due to just one single chemical constituent, as is often the case with "conventional" drugs. Rather, it is usually a mixture of constituents that are responsible for the therapeutic or protective effect of botanical medicines. Many of these herbal components are unique to a single plant species. They are not found anywhere else in nature, and have not yet been chemically identified. There are countless thousands of these herbal constituents called *phytochemicals* (from the Greek word for "plant").

Very few official methods are available for analyzing phytochemicals. Researchers were forced to develop qualitative and semi-quantitative chromatographic methods of separation and analysis in the painstaking attempt to unravel the complex chemical nature of botanicals.

So it was with the goji berry. The goal of scientists was to try to determine all of its biologically active principles, so that they could ascertain which of the many varieties of *Lycium* goji berries might be the most beneficial to humans.

The researchers knew that it might take many years to isolate and quantify every chemical constituent. However, they had an ingenious idea for a shortcut that would allow them to positively identify and catalog each type of berry, separating even those that appeared to be identical. Their solution was called *spectroscopic analysis*, a fingerprinting technique borrowed from the science of astrophysics.

CHAPTER 6

FINGERPRINTING THE GOJI BERRY: THE SPECIAL SIGNATURE

No two people on earth can have identical fingerprints. In fact, the chances of finding a match for even a portion of a finger-print are estimated at one in one quintillion (that's a one followed by 20 zeros), which explains why partial fingerprints are admitted as forensic evidence. Even identical twins do not share identical fingerprints. They may look similar, but they are easily distinguishable, even to a layman.

At this point, you might ask, "What does this have to do with goji berries? Goji berries don't have fingers."

This is true, but each variety does possess unique characteristics that distinguish it from any other type of goji berry. A berry from Ningxia may look and taste identical to one from Xinjiang, but in fact, they can be quite different when viewed through a *Fourier Transform Infrared Spectrometer.*

"A Fourier Transform What?"

Perhaps the best way to think of a spectrometer is to relate it to a prism. A prism takes the white light of the sun and breaks it up into its component colors of red, orange, yellow, green, blue, indigo and violet.

What we perceive as color is simply a reflection of the sun's energy in the narrow band of wavelengths and frequencies our eyes can see. In the same way that our ears cannot hear a high-pitched dog whistle, our eyes cannot detect any of the sun's rays that are outside their limited range.

To counter our built-in limitations, the military uses *night scopes*, which allow one to see the otherwise invisible, low-energy *infrared rays*.

On the other side of the visible spectrum, the use of a *black light* can allow one to see the fluorescent colors in the high-energy *ultraviolet* part of the spectrum.

There are other forms of energy as well. From lowest energy level to highest, the complete spectrum consists of radio waves, microwaves, infrared, visible light, ultraviolet, X-rays and gamma rays. Together, they are called the *electromagnetic spectrum*.

Everything You Ever Wanted to Know About Spectrometers

A spectrometer is an analytical device that is designed to measure how substances either absorb or reflect electromagnetic energy. Different spectrometers are specifically designed to work at different parts of the electromagnetic spectrum (i.e., a visible-light spectrometer measures how substances absorb or reflect visible light; an ultraviolet spectrometer works only in the UV range, etc.).

Perhaps this is as good a time as any to remind you that an apple is not really red. It's true! An apple only appears to be red because its skin absorbs the orange, yellow, green, blue, indigo and violet sunrays, but does not absorb the red ones. Like a mirror, it bounces the red light back to our eyes, and we say something clever such as, "that's a *red* apple."

If there were no red component to sunlight, an apple would appear to be black.

The Special Signature

If one were to put a truly red apple into a visible light spectrometer, one might see a graph like the one on the following page:

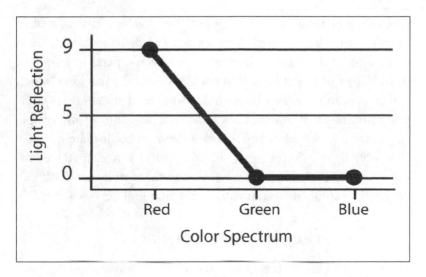

Apple Visible Light Special Signature

This graph is called the *visible light special signature* of the test apple. It is a measure of how light is being reflected or absorbed by the apple at the various wavelengths that make up the visible light part of the spectrum.

The peak on the graph above the word "red" shows that the apple is reflecting light at the red wavelengths, allowing it to be passed to a detector and recorded on the graph. The values of zero for green and blue waves demonstrate that the apple is absorbing those waves and not passing them through the machine to the detector.

Comparing Apples to Apples

In reality, no apple is a pure and uniform primary red. All apples contain colors other than red, so a true graph of an apple would be more complex than the one shown on page 19. The red peak would not be as high, and there would be peaks for other colors as well.

By the way, you can probably find a visible light spectrometer down at your local paint store. That's the machine that is used to match paint colors to target samples that you provide. Simply hand them a color chip, a swatch of fabric, or even a petal from one of Aunt Polly's prize petunias. They will put it in the machine, which will scan it and generate its visible light special signature. A computer program will convert the special signature into a paint recipe, and before you know it, you'll have a dead-on color match.

Visible light spectroscopy may be a perfect way to match paint, but it's woefully inadequate for the analysis of goji berries. It can only tell us color, and we already know that goji berries are red.

Properties More Valuable Than Color

Once we get outside the visible part of the electromagnetic spectrum, we can measure properties that are far more valuable than color. Of special interest is the *infrared* region, which can actually measure molecular bonding.

In FT-IR spectroscopy, radiation is passed through a sample of a goji berry. Some of the infrared radiation is absorbed by some of the molecules in the berry, and some of it is passed through or transmitted.

A highly sophisticated mathematical formula called the *Fourier Transform* is used in the analysis and interpretation of the data, with the result that a spectrum is generated that gives an incredibly detailed absorption and transmission fingerprint for the goji berry *at the molecular level.* It captures information about the atoms within the berry, the chemical bonds that hold the atoms together to form molecules, the nature of those molecules, and how they interact to pass energy from one to the other in the form of electron transfer.

Like any true fingerprint, the *FT-IR special signature* for each type of goji berry is unique. It can also tell the subtle differences between single-variety berries from neighboring valleys. More impressive still, it can discern differences between berries that were grown on the same vine in different years or under varying climate conditions.

The Goji Berry Roundup

Now armed with the FT-IR special signature technique, goji scientists began to collect samples of *Lycium* species from every well-known growing region throughout Asia: Ningxia, Xinjiang, Gansu, Tianjin Shi, Qinghai, Shanxi, Inner Mongolia, Sichuan and Tibet.

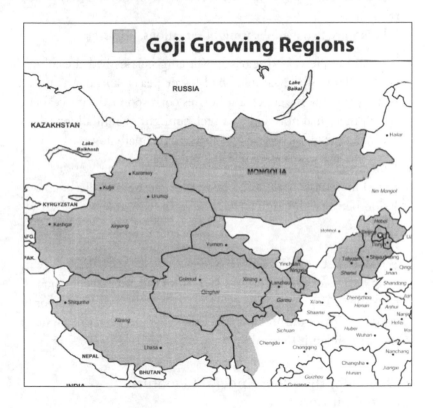

As they fed the berries into the spectrometer, an interesting pattern began to emerge. There seemed to be a great similarity between the special signatures of goji berries from each of these regions. That was to be expected, as all goji varieties have a close family resemblance. They are all of the *Lycium* genus.

There were several peaks, however, that varied greatly in height for different samples of berries. Special signature graphs of berries from Xinjiang and Ningxia tended to exhibit the highest peaks, with the rest of the samples showing peaks that were lower to varying degrees.

To the researchers, the discovery of these peaks indicated that there might be some unknown active compounds present in the goji berry, and that they were found in the famous berries of Ningxia and Xinjiang at higher levels than in the less renowned berries.

There were two complicating observations, however:

1. Not all samples of Ningxia or Xinjiang berries had these high peaks. Some of the samples had lower peaks, and it was noteworthy that the lower-testing berries corresponded with years in which there had not been as much sunlight or rainfall, or when late summer temperatures had been abnormally low.

2. Conversely, there were some samples from lesser regions that tested incredibly high, and once again there was a direct correlation between the high special peaks and an exceptional growing season.

But doesn't this make sense? Not every year is a "vintage" year, for goji berries or for fine wines. In fact, in the last 30 years, one of the premier vineyards in France has produced a "great" wine only three times. Twice during that time, the wine has been pronounced to be virtually unfit to drink!

In Search of the Ideal Special Signature for the Goji Berry

It had become obvious that the best goji berries were those with the highest peaks on their special signature graphs. Now it was time to find out what phytochemicals were responsible for those peaks.

Isolating the Active Principles

From information gleaned from the special signatures, scientists were able to determine the chemical nature of the unnamed active compounds in the goji berry. They did not know their exact structure, but they knew that they would be looking for *bioactive polysaccharides*, and that made them very excited.

Until recent years, scientists had lumped all polysaccharides together with other carbohydrates such as starches and sugars. They had considered them to be of value only as a source of energy. But that had all changed when it was discovered that certain types of polysaccharides could cause profound and beneficial changes in the human body.

What Are Bioactive Polysaccharides?

Bioactive polysaccharides, also called *proteoglycans*, are a family of complex carbohydrates that are bound to proteins. They are produced by some plants as an extremely effective defense mechanism against attack by viruses, bacteria, fungi, soil-borne parasites, cell mutations, toxic pollutants and environmental free radicals.

Fortunately for humans, many of these protective effects are conferred upon us when we eat plants that are rich in polysaccharides.

There are many types of bioactive polysaccharides, and they all seem to differ in their properties, health benefits and degrees of activity. Here are some of the areas currently under study:

Top Ten Benefits of Polysaccharides

1. Inhibit tumor growth

2. Prevent cancer

3. Neutralize the side effects of chemotherapy and radiation

4. Help normalize blood pressure

5. Help balance blood sugar

6. Combat autoimmune disease

7. Act as an anti-inflammatory

8. Balance immune function

9. Lower cholesterol and blood lipids

10. Increase calcium absorption

Although many plants produce small amounts of bioactive poly-saccharides, it seems that those with the highest levels of these protective compounds are those that are themselves most sorely in need of protection.

These polysaccharide-producing species include those that must attempt to survive under great stresses such as extremes of temperature, high altitude or wildly unpredictable precipitation.

No plant on earth grows under more stressful conditions than does the goji. It was not surprising, therefore, when scientists found the little red berry to be a treasure trove of highly bioactive polysaccharides.

The polysaccharides they found were different and more active than anything they had ever seen before.

CHAPTER 7

GOJI'S UNIQUE "MASTER MOLECULES"

Scientists determined their structural composition to be unique, peptide-bound acidic heteropolysaccharides of a type never before encountered in any of the world's tens of thousands of botanical species.

Four primary bioactive polysaccharides were discovered in *Lycium barbarum*. The scientists simply named them *Lycium barbarum polysaccharides* (abbreviated as LBP). Following the same logic, these four main polysaccharides were named LBP1, LBP2, LBP3 and LBP4.

LBP polysaccharides proved to be *glycoconjugates*, meaning that they are exceptional sources of the essential cell sugars—*rhamnose, xylose, glucose, mannose, arabinose* and *galactose*—that are necessary for proper immune function and intercellular communication. In fact, goji may be the richest source of glyconutrients yet found!

Research strongly suggests that goji's unique polysaccharides work in the body by serving as directors and carriers of the instructions that cells use to communicate with each other. In this way, it can be said that goji's LBP polysaccharides are "master molecules" by virtue of their ability to command and control many of the body's most important biochemical defense systems.

The Search Narrows

As the scientists began to retest their goji berry samples—this time looking for polysaccharide content—they found that there was great variation in levels of LBPs among the berries from different regions. The variations in LBP levels observed in any one sample corresponded exactly with the previously observed variations in special signature peak height for that same sample. In other words, good berries had high special peaks and high LBP content, whereas those with low peaks and low polysaccharides would be of little biological value.

CONCLUSION 1:
High special signature peaks = High levels of bioactive LBP polysaccharides = Potent goji berries

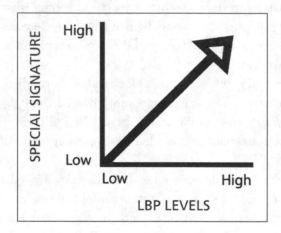

Berries that were said to be highly effective were, upon analysis, found to contain the full range of LBPs, not just one or two. Each of the four main polysaccharides has their own distinct benefits. Subsequent clinical studies would prove that all of the polysaccharides must be present for highest biological activity.

CONCLUSION 2:
All goji polysaccharides must be present for highest biological activity.

Also, it was found that the most highly prized berries from each region seemed to share the same balanced profile of LBPs. The "ordinary-grade" berries from Gansu and Ningxia might differ greatly from one another, but the very best berries from both places had a virtually identical polysaccharide composition.

This ideal balance of LBPs was seen most frequently in the berries of Xinjiang, followed very closely by those of Ningxia. Neither of these two goji capitals can produce world-class berries all the time, but now we know that, when they are at their best, they conform to an ideal LBP balance, which is shown on their special signature.

CONCLUSION 3:
All great goji berries share the same special signature.

This last conclusion was perhaps the most important. By the use of special signature fingerprinting techniques, it was now possible to judge the medicinal value of a goji berry by scientific means. All one needed to do was to test berries to see how well they stacked up against the "ideal" special signature of those from Xinjiang.

What Makes Xinjiang Berries So Ideal?

That's the question scientists were asking. Perhaps there was something about the extreme high altitude, the crystalline purity of the glacial water, the precipitous fluctuations of temperature, or some other factor that could explain the consistently high quality of Xinjiang goji berries. The biggest difference between Xinjiang and anywhere else seemed to be its situation in the shadow of the Heavenly Mountains, which we have previously described as being nearly the equal of the mighty Himalayas.

Interestingly, and quite coincidentally, our goji researchers had been recently contacted by a group of scientists from the Himalayas, who had inquired about special signature techniques. It seems they had discovered some rather remarkable properties of their own native goji berry, and they wanted to share data.

To the goji researchers, this came as quite a surprise. In their quest, they had not even considered berries from the Himalayas.

Nonetheless, they had been asked by the Himalayan group to perform special signature and LBP analysis. Graciously agreeing, they
awaited the arrival of samples.

The test results were simply astounding. The special signature
of the goji from the Himalayas was an exact match for the very best
Xinjiang and Ningxia berries. The polysaccharide value was sky-
high, with all LBPs in absolute perfect balance.

Ultimately the goji researchers came to understand and believe
that the true ancestral home of the goji berry was indeed the lofty
Himalayas.

They would learn how the goji plant had originated, and how it
had been dispersed around the world as the Himalayan people's
gift to the world.

CHAPTER 8

THE HIMALAYAS:
THE "ABODE OF SNOW"

When we think of the Himalayas, we might summon up images of breathtaking Mount Everest, the world's highest peak. Did you know that the Himalayas are still forming and that with every passing year, they actually increase in height? It's true, because the Himalayas are the result of a relatively recent collision between two continents (when we say *recent*, we're speaking in geological terms of thousands and thousands of years).

At the dawn of Creation, our planet was a far different place than the one we inhabit today. Instead of the seven continents that make up our modern world, the earth's ancient land masses were combined into two immense super-continents: *Eurasia* in the northern hemisphere, and *Gondwanaland* in the southern hemisphere.

During the Jurassic era, a substantial segment of Gondwanaland broke free and began to float slowly northward across the earth's surface toward Eurasia. Proceeding at the almost imperceptible pace of just *four inches per year*, the breakaway island forged onward until, with monumental force, it slammed into the southern end of the Eurasian continent.

Perhaps *slammed* is not the ideal choice of words for a collision taking place at four inches per year, but the force and momentum behind the collision was immense. Think of it as watching a high-speed head-on train wreck taking place in super-slow motion.

Nothing could stop the forward motion of the impinging island. It continued to push its massive weight aggressively against Eurasia, and the larger continent resisted stubbornly.

As the rock densities of both landmasses were similar, neither was able to subdue the other. Tremendous pressure mounted until, no longer able to be contained, it found relief in the only possible way, by thrusting the earth skyward along the entire 1,800–mile boundary between the battling continents.

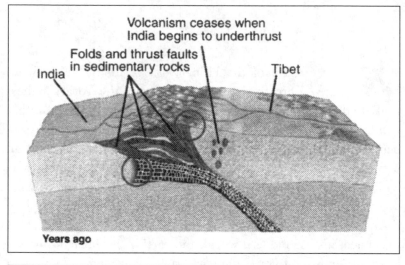

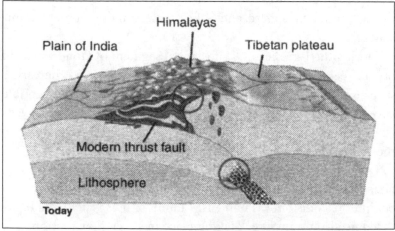

Formation of the Himalayas

Long buried layers of deep earth were upturned and sent soaring to heights of nearly 30,000 feet. The dramatic upheaval transformed the collision zone into an unbroken line of jagged peaks and steep canyons.

The newly formed mountain range welded the two land masses together. To the north, the plateau of Tibet extended into China. To the south of the mountains, the once-traveling island became what we now call the Indian subcontinent.

Remarkably, this collision isn't over yet. Even today, the Indian land mass is still plowing into Tibet at the breakneck speed of four inches per year, thrusting the Himalayan mountains ever higher. In fact the Himalayas are the world's youngest mountains!

At first, the new mountains and the lands surrounding them were virtually devoid of life. After all, had these majestic peaks not been there, the rain clouds sweeping up from the Indian Ocean would have passed over India into central Asia, leaving it a burning desert.

The skyscraping mountains did stop the clouds, the clouds brought the rains, and the rains transformed the barren crags into the snow-capped natural wonders that are today called the Himalayas (from the ancient Sanskrit for "abode of snow").

The Himalayan region has a climatic and geological diversity unlike anywhere else on earth. This is a land not only of lofty peaks and blue skies, but also of dense primeval forests, deep river gorges, verdant grasslands, cascading streams, and lush, fruit-laden valleys. Only here can one find the Alpine edelweiss thriving amongst tropical orchids. The native people have another name for this earthly paradise; one that requires no translation. They call it *Shangri-La*.

The soil of the Himalayas is incredibly rich in minerals upturned from deep within the earth during their formation. In fact, the region supports more than 18,440 species of exotic plants, many of which are found nowhere else on the planet.

Even more amazingly, the Himalayan people have found healing- and disease-preventive properties in more than 8,000 of their native plants. This great wealth of knowledge did not come overnight; it is a tradition that has been nurtured and passed along since the very beginnings of human civilization.

The Birthplace of Civilization

Archaeological evidence reveals that civilization first emerged in the valleys of the rivers coursing down from the Himalayan Mountains. When man elsewhere was cautiously emerging from his cave shelters, spectacular cities were flourishing in the fertile valleys of the Himalayas.

In the Indus River region, archaeologists have found evidence of man dating back thousands of years. We know also that, around 3,000 B.C., a great society developed in the Indus valley. This urban civilization flourished for nearly 1,500 years and was the world's first "melting pot."

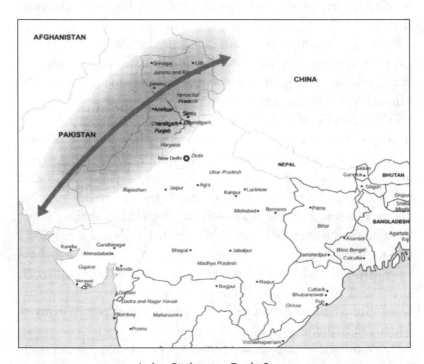

Indus Civilization Trade Route

Why were people drawn to the Himalayas from every corner of the world? One of the reasons for the rise and the prosperity of the Indus Civilization was its situation right along a natural trade route between central Asia and the Indian subcontinent.

Perhaps more important was that the Himalayas had become widely known as a serene and spiritual place, a land where all cultures were embraced and where all ideas were welcomed. It was this free interchange of ideas that led to the development of the world's first system of natural medicine.

The First Healers

The Traditional Himalayan Medicine System (THMS) has been passed down by word of mouth since the very beginning of civilization. Through their use of an extraordinary array of healing plants and the traditional methods that have been carefully developed over generations, Himalayan herbal practitioners have fought successfully against all types of diseases, conquering even those that we consider to be "incurable."

So successful were the ancient Himalayan healers that neighboring civilizations sent delegations to learn their secrets. It is said that the famous medical traditions of Tibet and China, and the Ayurvedic system of India all have their origins in THMS, and that they all owe a large debt to the unwritten teachings accumulated and handed down by generations of Himalayan practitioners.

Treating the Healthy Body to Prevent Illness

The Himalayan medicine system is more than merely a way of treating disease; it is also a prescription for healthy living. THMS is based upon a concept of wellness, of maintaining your strength and vitality, your mind and your spirit, so that disease cannot grab hold. That is why the most valuable medicinal plants in the Himalayan system are not those that cure disease. Rather, the most honored herbs are those that are taken when one is healthy and well, to help to prevent disease from occurring in the first place.

The concept of keeping the body healthy and disease-free sounds like good common sense, but it is in direct opposition to the big-money interests of our pharmaceutical-oriented Western system of medicine.

Our doctors, hospitals and drug companies have little interest in keeping us healthy. In fact, their very livelihood depends upon our being sick—as often as possible—so that we will require their very expensive services to put us back in good health.

A Himalayan healer would be saddened indeed to hear of how our modern medical system has corrupted the healing arts in the name of financial profit. He would be bewildered by our reliance on toxic chemotherapeutic agents, on risky surgical procedures, and on drugs that can have side effects exceeding any possible benefit.

Our close-minded doctors might simply dismiss Himalayan medicine as primitive and unsophisticated. The irony is that we are the primitive ones. How sophisticated can we be when our modern society is plagued by cancer, heart disease, high blood pressure, diabetes, arthritis, depression, sexual dysfunction, stroke, Alzheimer's disease and all types of degenerative and autoimmune diseases? In the Himalayas, these conditions are virtually unknown. To the contrary, these unassuming people are renowned for health and longevity unmatched anywhere on Earth.

CHAPTER 9

THE AMAZING PEOPLE
OF THE HUNZA VALLEY

The advent of the 20th century saw numerous British and European expeditions to the Himalayas. Some were Christian missions; yet others made perilous attempts to explore and chart the hundreds of unmapped mountains and remote valleys. In almost every case, explorers and missionaries returned home telling tales of an amazing race of mountain dwellers called the Hunzakuts. These residents of the fertile Hunza valley could perform unbelievable feats of strength and endurance, were able to scamper over cliffs with the agility of mountain goats, and could run for up to 60 miles at a stretch on narrow mountain passes without ever becoming tired or breathless. More amazingly, they could perform these feats well into an extraordinarily old age, with many of them living happily for more than 100 years!

Stories of the fabled Hunzakuts were reaching Europe just as a small group of forward-thinking doctors were exploring the relationship between a people's environment and their subsequent health.

London physician Dr. G. T. Wrench was one of these remarkable men. Years ahead of modern ecologists, Dr. Wrench had tried repeatedly to warn that improper use of the environment could have a tremendous negative impact on health. Wrench proposed that modern farming methods could lead only to destruction of the soil, loss of health and degradation of humans, while peasant farming systems are perpetual and health-producing. This had led him to study the Hunza people, whose advanced and sustainable irrigation techniques were allowing them to reap bountiful harvests from a land with an annual rainfall of less than 25.4 cm, or 10 inches.

Wrench's warnings were largely ignored, but the Hunzakuts fascinated European society. This prompted further expeditions by health researchers and government officials. In 1938, Dr. Wrench chronicled these expeditions to the Hunza valley in his book, *The Wheel of Health: The Study of a Very Healthy People:*

> *"The travelers and officials with one voice bear testimony to the Hunzakuts' physique. They find these people not only fearless, good-tempered and cheerful, but also possessing a marvelous agility and endurance.*
>
> *"They are a virile and cheerful people who persist in remaining free from disease, and are unsurpassed in health by any other nation in the world.*
>
> *"They are still a people peculiarly themselves. They have preserved their remoteness from the ways and habits of the modern world, and with it those methods of life which contribute or cause the excellent physique and bodily health which is theirs."*

Longevity Secrets of the Hunza People

Dr. Wrench attributes the remarkable health and longevity of the Hunzakuts in part to the distinctive qualities of the Himalayan soil. But as another important factor, he cites their uniquely healthful diet, which consists mainly of fruits. But these are not ordinary fruits; Himalayan fruits are remarkable for two reasons:

1. They capture from the soil the full spectrum of nutrients that were upturned from deep within the earth during the formation of the Himalayas. In the fruit itself, these essential nutrients are naturally chelated to fruit acids, which increases their bioavailability.

2. They are allowed to achieve full natural ripeness in the gentle

warmth of the golden Himalayan sun. Nowhere on earth is closer to the sun than the lofty Himalayas. This powerful exposure to the sun is more important than you might think.

The Schomberg Effect

Describing the relationship between the Himalayan sun and the unique properties of the fruit of the Hunza valley, Dr. Wrench speaks of the work of the noted British explorer Colonel Reginald Schomberg (1880–1958), who in 1936 made this original and important observation:

> "... there is such a direct relationship between the sun and fruit. Fruit, more obviously than other foods, ripens and colors in the sun. Sunlight is the carrier of the sun's quality. Through it that quality comes direct from the great orb of our being. It stores itself in sunbathed food, as in a minor way electricity is stored in a battery. The eating of fruit releases the sun's quality in its most direct and least interfered-with form."

This was a groundbreaking concept—fruit on the tree serving as "storage batteries" for the life-giving qualities of the sun, releasing the sun's goodness when the fruit is eaten.

The unfortunate thing for Schomberg is that he never presented his theory in a scientific treatise, but merely described it in the notebooks of his Himalayan expeditions. Consequently, his scientific observations went undiscovered for many years until they were recently unearthed.

Today, scientists are learning how to quantify the ability of living plants to absorb and retain the vital energy of the sun. These precise measurements also allow them to predict just how effectively and efficiently that energy might be transferred to us when we eat those plants. They call this determination of energy transfer potential the *Schomberg effect*. Simply put, foods with a high Schomberg effect can keep us healthier by facilitating the transfer of energy.

The Body Electric: A Shocking Tale

All matter is made up of atoms, and all atoms contain negatively charged high-energy particles called *electrons*. We know the term electron because of the word *electricity*, which is defined as a continuing handoff of *electrons* from one atom to a neighboring one that doesn't have enough.

Electric current moving through a copper wire is very much like a bucket brigade, or, better still, a game of hot potato. Each copper atom receives an electron from its neighbor, and just can't wait to dump it off onto the next poor atom down the line until someone turns off the switch and the circuit goes dead.

Why do atoms want to lose electrons so readily? Nobel laureate Dr. Albert Szent-Gyorgyi proposed that the essence of life is that the organic molecules in the body must be maintained in a state of electron desaturation. Szent-Gyorgyi tells us that only dead tissue has a full complement of electrons, while live tissue maintains a deficit of electrons.

Szent-Gyorgyi asserts that energy exchange, life's most important form of cellular communication, can only occur when there is a natural flow of electrons, a biological form of electricity, coursing throughout the body. All of the body's functions are directed, controlled and regulated by this flow of electricity.

Health exists when there is smooth flow of electrons, illness encroaches when the flow is significantly restricted, and death occurs when the energy transfer from this electron flow stops.

The Search for the Himalayan Longevity Fruit

Armed with testing methods for the Schomberg effect, researchers recently began to analyze the fruits that make up a good proportion of the Hunza diet. They did this with the aim of determining which ones might be the most responsible for the extreme good health and longevity of the Hunzakuts.

The fruits of the Hunza valley have been documented since 1899, when Lord Curzon made a visit there shortly before his appointment as viceroy. He described the orchards in the valley, their "rich spoil of apricots, walnuts, apples, pears, melons, mulberries, peaches, and grapes."

The researchers' opinion? Lord Curzon may have given us a great recipe for a fruit salad, but not a prescription for eternal youth. The Schomberg effect of these fruits is simply too low.

Still believing that Dr. Wrench and Colonel Schomberg were correct in their theory that a native fruit might hold the key to Hunza longevity, the researchers made the bold decision to broaden their search to include not just everyday fruits such as apricots and grapes, but medicinal ones as well.

Thus began a study of all 8,000 therapeutic plants in the Himalayan *Materia Medica*. Eliminating all roots, leaves, tree barks and herbs, they focused their attention solely on medicinal fruits until, at long last, they found their answer growing on a slender climbing vine. Their search had led them to a tiny red berry, a variant of *Lycium barbarum* known as goji. When they tested this goji, they were astounded. The Schomberg effect measured off the scale.

Moreover, as they continued to research goji, they soon found that they had not just uncovered some ordinary medicinal herb. To the contrary, they began to realize that the goji that originated in the Himalayas might well be the most powerful and important natural health discovery ever made.

CHAPTER 10

GOJI: A HIMALAYAN ORIGINAL

It is said that the goji vine has flourished in the Himalayan valleys since the beginning of time. The folks in Ningxia may not like it, but the goji from the Himalayas is the true original.

We are not certain how goji got its name, but it has been suggested that it takes its name from Gojal, the part of the Himalayas that borders the Hunza valley.

Regardless of the origin of the name, what is certain is that the ancient Himalayan herbal practitioners shared their secrets with the Chinese, Tibetans, Indians and others. Those who came to learn took the goji home with them and planted it in their own valleys.

Another sign that the goji from the Himalayas is the original is that it contains every desirable trait, in perfect balance. Its polysaccharide content is outstanding, its special signature is ideal, and it is a perfect receptacle for storing and transferring the energy of the sun, as measured by its extraordinarily high Schomberg effect.

"Where Can I Get Goji Berries of Himalayan Origin?"

The sad truth is that you can't. There just aren't enough to go around. Goji vines are not cultivated in the Himalayas; they simply grow in the wild, often in the most inaccessible places.

"So Your Suggestion Is . . . ?"

When you put this book down, I'm hoping you'll want to try goji berries. I'm certain that you can purchase dried berries on the Internet, but by doing so, you may be buying a product that will most likely not conform to the excellent special signature of the world's best berries, will not be standardized to a high level of perfectly balanced polysaccharides, and will not be tested for its Schomberg effect.

I would suggest that you reject such products and seek out a goji product that meets the demanding criteria that I have outlined in this book. A great goji berry product will meet the special signature profile of the goji of Himalayan origin, even if the berry is not from the Himalayas. For example, at various times, the berries of Xinjiang, Ningxia and other growing regions are of a quality sufficiently high to meet the established Himalayan special profile.

Remember, all goji berries came originally from the Himalayas. There are now dozens of varieties of berries growing in many countries, but the only ones that should rightfully be called the *true goji* are those which have retained the exact special signature and balanced polysaccharides of the original.

Therefore, when you're looking for goji berries, be demanding.

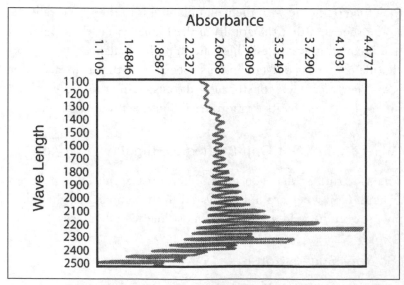

Ideal Special Signature

CHAPTER 11

SUGGESTED GOJI USAGE
FOR GOOD HEALTH

For everyday good health, start with a three-quarter dropper-ful (0.62 ml) or six sprays of the 100% goji berry extract twice daily. Many people will notice positive effects quickly, often within a matter of a few days. To achieve maximum benefit, however, you should allow a full six months of use, so that goji juice may work to bring your body back to the perfectly balanced state known to physicians as homeostasis.

Listen to your body. If, after the first month of use, you feel that your results are suboptimal, you may increase your daily dose to twelve sprays twice daily of the 100% goji berry extract per day. Remain at the twelve sprays twice daily dosage level for a full week, and, if necessary, add an additional ounce (30 ml) the following week. You can increase to $1^1/_2$ dropperfuls up to three times daily. You may take your daily serving all at once, or you may split it into as many portions as you like.

Goji juice is a food, so there is no danger of toxicity. However, you should always consult your physician or health advisor before starting to take any dietary supplement.

Special Needs

In the following 13 chapters and appendix, I will cover specific con-ditions in detail for which there exists a record of long and safe traditional use of goji, or for which there is compelling evidence of scientific or clinical efficacy. You will be provided with a brief overview of the condition, its believed causes, recommended life-style changes, and information on how a *high-quality* goji product can help. (Note: Some of the traditional and clinical literature refers to the use of fresh berries, whereas other resources cite dried berries. Many of the recent clinical studies have been carried out with either crude polysaccharide extracts or with isolated poly-saccharides. For your convenience, I have converted all of these into their equivalent dose of *high quality* 100% goji berry extract.)

In addition, the Appendix provides information on the usual dosage level for several other conditions for your convenience.

Every day, more and more research is emerging on this amazing little red berry, and I am committed to keeping you informed. In fact, it will be hard for me to update this book with new editions given the vast number of studies emerging on goji—but I will certainly try my best to do just that!

CHAPTER 12

ALLERGIES

You may not realize it, but your body is under constant attack by outside forces. Normally, your immune system responds to hostile foreign invaders—such as bacteria and viruses—by painting them with specific proteins called antibodies. These antibodies act as beacons, signaling specialized immune cells to rush to the site of infection so that they can disarm and destroy the attackers before they can cause harm to the body.

Sometimes, this same series of reactions is inexplicably triggered by harmless, everyday substances. This condition is known as an allergy, and the offending substance is called an allergen. Each time you come in contact with an allergen, certain cells in the body release chemical substances (such as histamine and leukotrienes), which results in one or more of the symptoms we associate with allergy such as: redness, swelling, itchy eyes, runny nose and breathing difficulties.

However, other lesser-known symptoms can include: absent-mindedness, anaphylaxis, asthma, burning eyes, constipation; coughing, depression, dermatitis, diarrhea, difficulty swallowing, distraction, dizziness, eczema, flushing, headaches, heart palpitations, impaired sense of smell, irritability/behavioral problems, itchy skin, joint aches, muscle pains, nasal polyps, nausea, postnasal drainage (postnasal drip), rapid pulse, shortness of breath, skin rashes, sleep difficulties, throat hoarseness, tingling nose, tiredness, vertigo, vomiting, and wheezing. This abnormal immune response is termed an allergic reaction.

The primary causes of allergy include ingestants (substances that enter the body by mouth such as food and drugs), inhalants (protein substances breathed in through the nose or mouth, such as pollen, mold spores, animal dander and house dust mites), and contact allergens that enter the body through the skin, such as powders, lotions, fragrances, some metals, latex, household cleaners and soap residue.

Other non-specific factors that may aggravate an allergy include changes in humidity, temperature (especially cold), infections and secondhand smoke.

It is important to remember that an allergy is not a result of either overactive or sluggish immune function; it is caused by immune abnormalities. Fortunately, traditional Asian medicine has long demonstrated that abnormal immune response can be treated successfully, without the need for harsh drugs.

In Asia, the goji berry has been used as a primary allergy therapy for centuries. The noted ethnobotanist Dr. James A. Duke classifies goji as an immunomodulator—an enhancing substance that can balance and normalize abnormal immune response.

In a study of goji berry reported in the *Journal of the Beijing Medical University* (1992), it was noted that goji reduced antibodies associated with allergy-type reactions, which was presumed to be accomplished through the mechanisms of promoting CD8(+) T-cells and regulating cytokines. Probably as a result of this activity, goji berry has also been reported to be a useful treatment for psoriasis.

In a review of research appearing in *Recent Advances in Chinese Herbal Drugs*, Dr. Zhou Jinhuang points out that goji's master molecule polysaccharides enhance cell-mediated and humoral immune responses, increasing normal activity of T-cells, cytotoxic T-cells and natural killer cells.

Usual dosage level: For all allergic conditions, research suggests a daily usage of $1^1/_2$ dropperfuls, or twelve sprays, twice to three times daily of 100% goji berry extract, taken with meals.

CHAPTER 13

ANTI-AGING

Old age may be inevitable, but it doesn't have to be accompanied by a loss of health and vigor. With a little motivation, you can control, delay and even reverse many of the degenerative processes of aging.

There are many theories on aging, but the most prominent one asserts that our modern lifestyle is to blame. Chronic exposure to environmental toxins, pollutants and carcinogens causes damage to DNA, the body chemical responsible for the exact duplication of healthy cells. Damaged DNA may produce mutant cells that, as they accumulate, can impair the function of the body's tissues and vital organs.

DNA is the most important chemical in your body, carrying the blueprint of your entire genetic history. Goji's betaine and master molecule polysaccharides can restore and repair damaged DNA, protecting your body's ten trillion cells.

One cannot die merely of old age. Your ultimate demise is caused, not by advancing age itself, but by the diseases and degenerative conditions that accompany it. The good news is that many of these diseases can be prevented or controlled by the daily use of the goji berry.

Dozens of modern scientific studies have confirmed goji's reputation in Asia as the "longevity fruit." Its unique master molecule polysaccharides, powerful antioxidants and unsurpassed nutrient density help your body to initiate and sustain a strong and multi-faceted defense against aging.

Also, as an adaptogen, goji helps the body to adapt and to cope with stress—a prime factor in the aging process. It also provides the energy reserves to help you handle just about any difficulty, and goji's unique polysaccharide complex has been found to be a powerful secretagogue (a substance that stimulates the secretion of rejuvenative human growth hormone by the pituitary gland).

Brain cells are also susceptible to the aging process. Particularly, they are extremely sensitive to oxygen deficiency, which cause deficits in cognition, memory, recall ability and other brain function. Free radical activity and low levels of choline are major factors in Alzheimer's disease. Goji's unique master molecule polysaccharides and powerful antioxidants and choline precursors fight the free radical damage associated with Alzheimer's disease. Goji also increases the body's production of an enzyme that inhibits lipid peroxidation, the cause of myelin loss (the protective coating on nerves).

Finally, goji's flavonoids protect against narrowing of the arteries, keeping them open so they can deliver oxygen and nutrients to brain cells. Zhang (1993) studied the role of goji's unique LBP polysaccharides in fighting peroxidation, a primary cause of premature cell death.

Usual dosage level: To fight aging, research suggests a usage of $1^1/_2$ dropperfuls of high quality 100% goji berry extract taken twice daily at mealtime. Two ounces of goji juice can be taken twice daily if the extract is not available.

CHAPTER 14

ARTHRITIS

The incidence of arthritis is increasing at an alarming rate. According to statistics published by the Arthritis Foundation, the number of Americans with arthritis or chronic joint symptoms has doubled since 1985 and now affects one in three adults.

The most common form of arthritis—the "wear and tear" degenerative condition known as osteoarthritis (OA)—is most often seen in people over 60. However, OA is not the only form of arthritis. Although many of us refer to it as if it were a single disease, arthritis is actually a catchall term that covers more than 100 medical conditions, including: rheumatoid arthritis (RA)—caused when the immune system spirals out of control, attacking healthy joint cells as well as invading virus cells; systemic lupus; gout; ankylosing spondylitis—a type of arthritis in which inflammation causes the bones of the spine to grow together; juvenile arthritis (an umbrella term for all types of arthritis that occur in children); and scleroderma—a connective tissue disease that can cause extreme hardening of the skin, resulting in deposition of scar-like patches.

Arthritis can strike at any age, often without warning. In its various forms, arthritis affects more than 70 million adults and 300,000 children in America.

It has been estimated that there are more than 200 causes of the various forms of arthritis. And yet, there are some key risk factors. Cigarette smoking has been proven over and over again to increase the risk of rheumatoid arthritis. A recent large-scale study published in the *Annals of Rheumatic Diseases* concluded that even moderate smokers (six per day) could increase their risk by as much as 1,500%! Obesity is another major cause of arthritis. According to an article in the *American Journal of Clinical Nutrition*, the single biggest risk factor for osteoarthritis in the hips and hands of people older than 60 is being overweight. Reducing the symptoms of this painful disease should be a great inspiration to drop those pounds.

No matter what the source of arthritis, there is always the common factor of joint inflammation, often accompanied by pain, stiffness, restricted motion, warmth, swelling, and damage to the protective joint cartilage and surrounding tissues. This damage becomes progressively debilitating as joints become weakened and destabilized. Ultimately, arthritis can turn even the simplest daily tasks into a painful ordeal.

For those diagnosed with systemic forms of arthritis, the situation can be far worse. Systemic arthritis can affect the whole body, wreaking havoc on the heart, lungs, kidneys, blood vessels and skin.

Whether instigated by tobacco smoke, obesity, genetics, stress or other factors, all forms of arthritis are marked by chronic inflammation, which is caused by the body's overproduction of inflammatory prostaglandins (such as PGE-2) and enzymes (such as COX-2). These dangerous body chemicals cause the generation of free radicals, which act like 'mini-grenades' that can detonate anywhere in the body, causing irreparable damage.

The inflammatory free radical most often implicated in arthritis is known as superoxide. Under normal conditions, the body is able to keep superoxide in check by producing the enzyme superoxide dismutase (SOD) to intercept and neutralize it before it can cause pain, inflammation and cell damage.

Extensive scientific research over the past 20 years has shown that in acute and chronic inflammation, superoxide is produced at a rate that overwhelms the capacity of the body's SOD enzyme defense system to remove it. Such an imbalance can only result in significant damage.

Protective and beneficial roles of SOD have been clinically

demonstrated in arthritis and other inflammatory diseases. These results prove the concept that superoxide has an important role in human disease and that their removal by SOD does in fact result in beneficial outcomes.

One study in China found that the ingestion of goji resulted in a remarkable 40 percent increase of this extremely important anti-inflammatory enzyme. In addition, more than 40 years of research have revealed goji's ability to regulate immunity. Acting as an adaptogen, it can help to increase low immune function. Goji can also help to quiet a hyperactive immune system, bringing it back to a more normal level. Goji can also help with significant weight loss— an important factor in preventing and managing arthritis.

Usual dosage level: For all arthritic conditions, research suggests a maintenance usage of $1\frac{1}{2}$ dropperfuls, or twelve sprays of 100% goji berry extract, two to three times per day at mealtime. During times of flare-ups, the serving size may be doubled.

CHAPTER 15

ATHLETIC PERFORMANCE

All athletic activities are competitive by nature. This is readily observed in team sports, or in a casual one-on-one game of basketball or golf. Yet, even a solo athletic event is a competition that pits you against your own personal best.

Competitive athletes are constantly searching for ways to gain an advantage over opponents. The desire for an "edge" exists in all sports, at all levels of play. Successful athletes rely on practice and hard work to increase their skill, speed, power and ability. Many also find a competitive edge by enlisting trainers or using the latest high-tech equipment.

There are many healthy ways to increase your strength or improve your performance. The National Institutes of Health suggest that you keep the following tips in mind: Train safely, without using drugs; eat a healthy diet; get plenty of rest; set realistic goals and be proud of yourself when you reach them; seek out training supervision, coaching and advice from a reliable professional; and avoid injuries by playing safely and using protective gear.

Another safe and healthy way to enhance athletic performance is the use of certain rare plants and herbs called adaptogens. Adaptogens work by helping the body to adapt to changes and stress, without side effects or dangers.

Although knowledge of adaptogens has been with us since antiquity, the term *adaptogen* itself is relatively new; Russian scientists coined it during the Soviet era of Olympic athletic dominance.

Dr. Sergey Portugalov, chief advisor in nutrition and pharmacology to the Russian Olympic teams and an expert member of the World Anti-Doping Association (WADA), has recently made this candid admission: "Sports have always been a major priority in Russia—and now the world will know what has helped us achieve domination. Hundreds of researchers secretly worked to improve training and nutrition, which we consider fundamental for elite athletes. For the past ten years, we have primarily focused on achieving results without using drugs. Our greatest competitive advantage came from performance supplements derived from natural plant materials (adaptogens). The nutritional support provided by these supplements helped our athletes achieve better performance, stamina, endurance, strength, recovery, immune resistance, muscle development and adaptation to changes in climate, time zones and altitude. The world has seen the results at the last four Olympic Games. But until recently our revolutionary discoveries were a closely guarded secret."

Adaptogens significantly improve all parameters of exercise capacity, including maximal oxygen consumption (VO2 max), tolerance and fatigue threshold. They increase energy, endurance and vitality. They help fight the damaging effects of stress that result when the adrenal glands overproduce cortisol, a muscle-wasting, catabolic (protein-destroying) hormone. They promote cardiovascular health and help to strengthen your heart and circulation, allowing you to perform with less demand on your cardiovascular resources. They assist in recovery from intense workouts by enhancing the body's replenishment of the two important muscle fuels (glycogen and creatine phosphate)—both of which are depleted during exercise—thus enabling you to avoid 'burnout' associated with glycogen depletion and allowing you to fit more high-quality workouts into a defined period. They enhance mental alertness by improving reflex response, reaction time, attention span, hearing, eyesight and motor coordination. They promote more efficient oxygen use—your muscle and brain cells require oxygen in order to produce energy. They also improve circulation and increase the capacity of cells to uptake and utilize oxygen, and protect your body's most important organ for detoxification and tissue repair—your liver—which can be stressed during processing of the metabolic wastes produced by vigorous exercise. Adaptogens also enhance endocrine function by strengthening the activity of the glands most responsible for energy, muscle growth and repair (adrenal, thymus, thyroid, pituitary and hypothalamus). Last but certainly not least, they stimulate muscle regeneration through steroid-free anabolic action.

In Asia, no adaptogen is more revered than goji. The fruit is held in such high regard that it has been named a supertonic (a substance that harmonizes the structures and functions of the entire body). Goji increases exercise tolerance, stamina and endurance, and helps to eliminate fatigue, especially when you are recovering from injury or illness.

Goji's unique master molecule polysaccharides also help prevent sore muscles by increasing activity of the lactic-acid-removing enzyme lactate dehydrogenase. It also accelerates clearance of blood urea nitrogen, a toxin produced during exercise. And, as Asia's premier adaptogen, goji helps the body to adapt and to cope with stress, providing the energy reserves to help you handle just about any difficulty.

Goji also stimulates the release by the pituitary gland of hGH, the youth hormone. The benefits of hGH are extensive and include production of lean muscle, reduction of body fat, better sleep, improved memory, accelerated healing and much more.

Finally, goji helps protect and preserve your hard-won gains in the gym by helping to restore and repair damaged DNA, protecting each of your body's trillions of muscle cells.

Usual dosage level: For athletic performance enhancement, research suggests a daily usage of $1^1/_2$ dropperfuls, or twelve sprays twice daily of high-quality 100% goji berry extract, taken in divided doses before and after exercise.

CHAPTER 16

CHILDREN'S HEALTH

Keeping your children healthy is not an easy task. Colds, flu and other contagious diseases often spread with lightning speed and children tend to be the most vulnerable. Unlike adults, young children may not have been exposed to many common germs. Their immune systems may not have had the chance to develop resistance to infection.

And yet, some children appear to have a greater natural resistance to contagious diseases. These are the lucky kids who either do not get sick or always seem to bounce back quickly whenever they do catch a bug.

The good news is that you can help your children to be one of the "lucky" ones by following a few healthy guidelines. Eating well and being physically active are keys to your child's well-being. Not only will this help to keep them well when they're young, it will also build up their resistance to disease and protect them later in life. First and foremost, eliminate secondhand smoke. According to Dr. Beverly Kingsley of the Centers for Disease Control and Prevention, cigarette smoke contains more than 4,000 toxins. Kids are more susceptible than adults to the harmful effects of secondhand smoke. It increases a child's risk of SIDS, bronchitis, ear infections and asthma. It may also affect intelligence and neurological development. Enforce regular sleep—many older children, especially high-school students, are sleep-deprived. Irregular sleep reduces activity of natural killer cells, a key immune function. Parents should help their children plan schedules that permit eight to ten hours of sleep per night.

Here are some additional tips for parents:

- Make sure your child eats breakfast. This meal provides children with the energy they need to listen and learn in school.

- Offer your child a wide variety of foods such as grains, vegetables, fruits, low-fat dairy products and lean meat or beans.

- Talk with your healthcare provider if you are concerned about your child's eating habits or weight.

- Cook with less fat. Bake, roast or poach foods instead of frying.

- Limit the amount of added sugar in your child's diet.

- Involve your child in planning and preparing meals. Children may be more willing to eat the dishes they help make.

- Be a role model for your children. If they see you being physically active and having fun, they are more likely to be active and stay active throughout their lives.

- Encourage your child to be active every day and involve the whole family in activities.

Finally, make sure your kids get goji every day. One of the most beneficial uses of goji is its ability to strengthen the immune system to protect your child against disease. In traditional Asian medicine, the goji berry is renowned as an adaptogen, meaning that it has a rare ability to help your child to adapt to adverse conditions. In dozens of laboratory and clinical studies, goji has been shown to boost immune function. With daily use, it supports the body's own processes to maintain peak health and prevent development of disease.

Usual dosage level: For growing children, research suggests a daily usage of $1^1/_2$ dropperfuls, or twelve sprays of high-quality 100% goji berry extract, twice daily, taken with meals or before exercise or play activities.

CHAPTER 17

DEPRESSION

A depressive disorder is an illness that involves the body, mood and thoughts. It affects the way you eat and sleep, the way you feel about yourself and the way you think about things. A depressive disorder is more than just feeling sad, "blue" or "down in the dumps." People with a depressive illness cannot merely "pull themselves together" and get better. Without treatment, symptoms can last for weeks, months or years. Appropriate treatment, however, can help most people who suffer from depression.

The following are the most common symptoms of depression. If you experience five or more of these symptoms for two weeks or longer, you may be depressed:

- Sadness, anxiety or "empty" feelings

- Decreased energy, fatigue or being "slowed down"

- Loss of interest or pleasure in activities that were once enjoyed, including sex

- Insomnia, oversleeping or waking much earlier than usual

- Loss of weight or appetite, or overeating and weight gain

- Feelings of hopelessness and pessimism

- Feelings of helplessness, guilt and worthlessness

- Difficulty concentrating, making decisions or remembering

- Restlessness, irritability or excessive crying

- Chronic aches and pains or physical problems that do not respond to treatment

- Thoughts of death, suicide or suicide attempts

According to National Institute of Mental Health statistics, nearly 20 million American adults suffer from a depressive illness. It is twice as common in women as in men; 10–25 percent of American women and 5–12 percent of men will become clinically depressed at some point in their lives.

There are many roots of depressive conditions. Some types of depression run in families, occurring generation after generation. Studies have also suggested that depression may be associated with chemical imbalances in the brain, especially of the hormone serotonin. Life events can trigger depression as well—job loss, retirement, divorce, death of a loved one, or moving to a new house can precipitate a depressive illness. And depression tends to strike those who are living alone, in isolation, or without a support network of close friends or family. Those with life-threatening or long-term physical illness such as cancer, stroke, arthritis or heart disease are vulnerable to depression. And sometimes, even personality can play a part—people with low self-esteem, who consistently view themselves and the world with pessimism, or who are easily overwhelmed by stress, are prone to depression.

Depression treatment usually consists of antidepressant medication—which can be effective, but typically has side effects, and non-drug therapy. Often a combined treatment is used: medication to gain relatively quick relief and psychotherapy to learn more effective ways to deal with life stresses. Relaxation therapy and support groups are also utilized.

If you suffer from depression, there are some things you can do to help yourself:

- Don't bottle things up. Try to talk to someone close to you. It helps to have a good cry and talk things through.

- Don't set unrealistic or difficult goals for yourself. Depression tends to make you think in terms of "all or nothing." Resist and just do what you can.

- Keep yourself occupied as much as possible in ways that keep you from thinking too much.

- Get exercise if you can. The results of the physical exertion will lift your depression temporarily at least, in addition to the other benefits of exercise.

- Do some light activities or get out of the house for some fresh air. It helps to take your mind off your troubles.

- Eat a balanced diet, although you may not feel like eating.

- Maintain a regular sleep pattern, aiming for at least seven hours per night. Do not sleep in, even if you feel exhausted in the morning. Set a time to get up every morning and get out of bed.

- Do not drown your sorrows in alcohol. It may give immediate relief, but alcohol ultimately depresses your mood. It is also bad for your health.

- Don't despair: Remind yourself that many other people have suffered from depression and have become better. With treatment, you will eventually improve, just like they did.

In Asia, goji has enjoyed a long and well-deserved reputation as an energizing supertonic. Known as the "happy berry," goji has a legendary ability to promote cheerfulness and brighten the spirit. In fact, it has been noted that the only known side effect of goji is that continued consumption may make it impossible for you to stop smiling!

Goji offers a host of unique benefits that should be of great interest to anyone fighting depression. As an adaptogen, it helps the body to adapt to and cope with stress and provides the energy reserves to help you handle just about any difficulty. Goji also fights fatigue and boosts stamina, while improving sleep quality. In several medical study groups with elderly people, nearly all patients taking goji reported better quality of sleep.

Usual dosage level: For depressive disorders, research and traditional use suggest a daily intake of $1^1/_2$ dropperfuls, or twelve sprays, two to three times daily, of high-quality 100% goji berry extract.

CHAPTER 18

DIABETES

The World Health Organization has declared diabetes to be the world's fastest growing disease, describing it as "the silent epidemic." There are 194 million people worldwide with diabetes—more than 18 million people in the United States alone, of which nearly one-third are undiagnosed. This can be devastating, as diabetes is the main cause of kidney failure, limb amputation, and new onset blindness in American adults. People with diabetes are also two to four times more likely than people without diabetes to develop heart disease. In fact, 65 percent of diabetics die from a heart attack or stroke.

Diabetes is a disorder that affects the way your body deals with the foods you eat. Normally, carbohydrate foods are broken down into the sugar glucose, which travels in the blood (hence the name blood sugar) until it reaches your cells, where it is taken in and used for growth and energy. For this to happen, however, the hormone insulin must be present. Produced by the pancreas, insulin acts as a key that unlocks cells so that they can receive blood glucose. In diabetes, either the pancreas may produce insufficient insulin, or the body has lost its ability to use it effectively (insulin resistance). Glucose builds up in the blood, overflows into the urine, and passes out of the body without fulfilling its role as the body's main source of fuel.

Unfortunately, anyone can become diabetic at any time, but you may have an increased risk of getting diabetes if you are

45 years old or older; are overweight; are of African, Hispanic, Asian, Mediterranean, Pacific Island or Native American descent; have a parent, brother or sister with diabetes; have high blood pressure (above 140/90); have low HDL (good cholesterol) and high levels of blood fats; had diabetes when pregnant or gave birth to a large baby (over 9 pounds); and/or are physically active less than three times a week.

Symptoms of diabetes include: extreme thirst; urinating frequently; feeling very hungry or tired; losing weight without trying; having sores that heal slowly; having dry, itchy skin; losing the feeling in your feet or having tingling in your feet; and having blurry eyesight.

There are four main kinds of diabetes: Type 1 diabetes affects approximately 5 percent of all diabetics and is usually first diagnosed in children or young adults. (Type 1 diabetics must take insulin, as the body no longer produces it.) Type 2 diabetes affects 90 to 95 percent of all diabetics, usually begins with insulin resistance, and is more likely in those who are overweight or inactive. Gestational diabetes affects some women during the late stages of pregnancy—although it usually goes away after the baby is born, a woman who has had it is more likely to develop type 2 diabetes later in life. Pre-diabetes is a condition in which blood glucose levels are higher than normal but not high enough for a diagnosis of type 2 diabetes.

A major study reported in the February 7, 2002, edition of the *New England Journal of Medicine* concluded that type 2 diabetes can be avoided with a combination of a low-fat diet, regular exercise (such as walking for 30 minutes, five times a week) and a modest weight reduction of just five to seven percent (10 to 14 pounds for a 200 pound person).

If you do have diabetes, there are simple steps you can take to manage it. The National Diabetes Education Program suggests that you reduce your risk of heart disease and stroke by working with your healthcare team to monitor three critical factors, which they have named the *Diabetic ABCs*. A is for the A1C test. (This is a number that shows how well your blood glucose has been controlled over the last three months and should be checked at least twice a year.) B is for blood pressure. The goal for most people is 130/80. And C is for cholesterol. Bad cholesterol (LDL) can oxidize and clog blood vessels, causing heart attack or stroke, while good cholesterol (HDL) helps to lower bad cholesterol. (The goal for most people is LDL under 100 and HDL over 40.) In addition, you should: follow your diabetes food plan; eat the right portions of healthy foods and eat foods that have less salt and fat; get 30 to 60 minutes of activity at least five days per week; stay at a healthy weight; stop smoking; check your feet every day for cuts, blisters, red spots and swelling; and call your healthcare team right away about any sores that won't heal.

Brush your teeth and floss every day. Get your vision checked regularly. And check your blood glucose the way your doctor tells you to.

Goji can also help. This tiny red fruit has been used in China for the treatment of diabetes for many years, and its polysaccharides have been shown to help balance blood sugar and insulin response. It also contains betaine, which can prevent fatty liver disease and vascular damage often seen in diabetics. Goji also assists in weight loss by enhancing the conversion of food into energy instead of fat, and it increases exercise tolerance, stamina and endurance.

Usual dosage level: Check with your health practitioner for dosage. 100% goji berry extract has no sugar, therefore it should be safe for diabetics.

CHAPTER 19

DIGESTIVE DISORDERS

You may be able to ignore a cold, a headache or a sore elbow, but a digestive problem is something else altogether. Whether it's gas, intestinal cramps, a bout of nausea or a chronic condition like irritable bowel syndrome, a gastrointestinal disorder commands your full attention. Some digestive conditions are merely annoying, but others, if left untreated, can affect the health of your entire body and can even become life-threatening.

Researchers have only recently begun to understand the many and often complex diseases that affect the digestive system. This area of scientific research is highly active, as digestive disorders affect so many people—an estimated 70 million Americans alone.

Every section of the GI (gastrointestinal) tract is prone to its own unique disorders. Fortunately, for all but a few, we now have simple treatments that will, at the very least, relieve the symptoms.

Gastroesophageal reflux disease (GERD) is caused by a backflow (reflux) of acid stomach contents into the esophagus, due to a weakness in the muscle that acts like a valve between the esophagus and stomach. When refluxed stomach acid touches the lining of the esophagus, it causes a burning sensation in the chest or throat (heartburn). The fluid may even be tasted in the back of the mouth. This is called acid indigestion. Symptoms usually occur within an hour after eating and are most likely to strike when you lie down, bend or stoop.

If you experience heartburn more than twice a week, you may

have GERD, and it can eventually lead to more serious health problems if left untreated. Antacids are effective for immediate relief. Many people with GERD are also overweight, and successful long-term solutions involve losing weight to reduce pressure on the abdomen. Other tips: avoid tight clothing, don't lie down until two to three hours after eating, and elevate the head of your bed by 30 degrees.

Eat smaller, more frequent meals, and forgo high-fat foods, caffeine, chocolate and smoking.

Gastroenteritis is an irritation and inflammation of the digestive tract. Its symptoms include abdominal pain, vomiting and diarrhea brought on by exposure to bacteria, amoebas, parasites, toxins, certain drugs, enzymes or allergens in foods. Treatment usually includes bed rest, fluids, bismuth-containing products such as Pepto-Bismol and anti-nausea drugs.

Gastritis is an inflammation of the stomach lining. Some people with gastritis have no symptoms, but many experience vague pain, a feeling of fullness, loss of appetite, belching, nausea and vomiting. Atrophic gastritis is a weakening of digestion caused by reduced activity of stomach cells. Treatment for gastritis consists of eliminating irritating foods, avoiding aspirin, and taking antacids if the condition persists.

Ulcers can occur almost anywhere in the esophagus, stomach or small intestine. Almost all stomach ulcers are caused either by a bacterial infection by Helicobacter pylori (H. pylori) or by use of NSAIDs (non-steroidal pain medications such as aspirin, ibuprofen or naproxen). Most H. pylori–related ulcers can be cured with antibiotics. NSAID-induced ulcers can be cured with time, stomach-protective medications, antacids and avoidance of NSAIDs.

Irritable bowel syndrome (IBS) involves a problem in the workings of the muscles in the intestines, which is characterized by gas, abdominal pain, and diarrhea or constipation, or both. Although it can cause considerable pain and discomfort, it does not damage the digestive tract, nor does it lead to more serious digestive diseases later. It occurs more frequently in women under age 35 and may be related to psychological stress. Treatment includes a diet high in fiber and low in fat. Certain gas-producing foods, such as those in the cabbage family, should be avoided, as should any other suspected irritants.

Crohn's disease is an uncomfortable inflammation of the digestive tract. It usually attacks the small intestine but can also be found anywhere along the entire digestive tract. Crohn's disease causes pain, cramping, tenderness, gas, fever, nausea and diarrhea, and is possibly caused by a hyperactive immune system.

Goji itself is easily digested, especially when taken in its highly bio-available juice form, and is helpful for all digestive disorders. It has long been used in the treatment of atrophic gastritis. As an adaptogen, it can also help the body to adapt and to cope with stress—often a factor in flare-ups for those with digestive disorders, including ulcers and IBS.

Goji also balances immune response. It is important to remember that an autoimmune disorder such as Crohn's disease is not a result of either overactive or sluggish immune function; it is caused by immune abnormalities. Fortunately, traditional Asian medicine has long demonstrated that abnormal immune response can be treated successfully, without the need for harsh drugs. In Asia, the goji berry has been used as an immune system regulator for centuries. The noted ethnobotanist Dr. James A. Duke classifies goji as an immunomodulator—an enhancing substance that can balance and normalize abnormal immune response.

Finally, as reported in the *Journal of the Beijing Medical University* (1992), goji reduces antibodies associated with allergy-type reactions, which can also trigger certain digestive disorders.

Usual dosage level: For all digestive disorders, research suggests a daily usage of $1^{1}/_{2}$ dropperfuls, or twelve sprays of high-quality 100% goji berry extract, taken with meals.

CHAPTER 20

FIBROMYALGIA

F ibromyalgia is a chronic disorder characterized by widespread muscle pain, fatigue and multiple tender points. The word is derived from the Latin term for fibrous tissue (*fibro*) and the Greek words for muscle (*myo*) and pain (*algia*). Tender points are specific places on the body—such as the neck, shoulders, back, hips, and upper and lower extremities—where people with fibromyalgia feel pain in response to slight pressure.

According to a paper published by the American College of Rheumatology (ACR), fibromyalgia affects three to six million Americans. Between 80 and 90 percent of those diagnosed with fibromyalgia are women, but men and children also can be affected. Most people are diagnosed during middle age, although the symptoms often become present earlier in life. People with certain rheumatic diseases—such as rheumatoid arthritis or lupus—may be more likely to have fibromyalgia. Several studies have indicated that women who have a family member with fibromyalgia are more likely to have it themselves.

Although the exact causes of fibromyalgia are unknown, a number of factors may be involved. Many people develop fibromyalgia in connection with stressful or traumatic events, automobile accidents, repetitive injuries or illness. For others, the condition seems to occur spontaneously with no apparent causative link.

Many researchers are examining other causes, including problems with how the central nervous system processes pain. According to this theory, people with fibromyalgia may have a genetic pre-disposition to react strongly to stimuli that most people would not perceive as painful.

Fibromyalgia can interfere with your ability to carry on normal daily activities. Like arthritis, fibromyalgia is considered a rheumatic condition (one that impairs the joints and/or soft tissues and causes chronic pain). Unlike arthritis, however, fibromyalgia does not cause inflammation or destruction of the joints.

In addition to pain and fatigue, people who have fibromyalgia may experience: sleep disturbances, morning stiffness, headaches, irritable bowel syndrome (IBS), painful menstrual periods, numbness or tingling of the extremities, restless leg syndrome (RLS), temperature sensitivity, and cognitive and memory problems (sometimes referred to as "fibro fog").

Unfortunately, there are currently no diagnostic laboratory tests for fibromyalgia. Standard laboratory tests fail to reveal a physiological reason for pain. Because of this, some doctors may wrongly conclude that your pain is "in your mind," or they may tell you there is little they can do. A doctor familiar with fibromyalgia, however, can make a diagnosis based on two criteria established by the ACR: a history of widespread pain lasting more than three months and the presence of eleven or more tender points on the body.

Fibromyalgia treatment often requires a team approach with your doctor, a physical therapist, possibly other health professionals, and most importantly, yourself, all playing an active role. You may find several members of the treatment team you need at a clinic. Some clinics deal specifically with pain management and others specialize in arthritis and other rheumatic diseases, including fibromyalgia.

At present, there are no medications approved by the U.S. Food and Drug Administration (FDA) for treating fibromyalgia. Doctors treat fibromyalgia with a variety of medications developed and approved for other purposes. These include analgesics (painkillers), nonsteroidal anti-inflammatory drugs (NSAIDs) and anti-depressants. Other symptom-specific medications include sleep medications, muscle relaxants and headache remedies.

People with fibromyalgia also may benefit from a combination of physical and occupational therapy, by learning pain management and coping techniques, and by properly balancing rest and activity. Many people also report varying degrees of success with holistic therapies including massage, Pilates method, chiropractic treatments, acupuncture and various dietary supplements.

There are many things you can do to minimize the impact of fibromyalgia on your life. These include: getting enough sleep and the right kind of sleep, which can help ease the pain and fatigue of fibromyalgia; exercising—it's crucial to be as physically active as possible—research has repeatedly shown that regular exercise is one of the most effective treatments for fibromyalgia; eating well—not only will proper nutrition give you more energy and make you generally feel better, it will also help you avoid other health problems.

Fortunately, goji can also help tremendously—and without the harmful side effects of drugs. Ranked as one of Asia's premier adaptogens, goji is known to fight fatigue and boost stamina, while increasing exercise tolerance, stamina and endurance. And in several medical study groups, nearly all patients taking goji reported better quality of sleep—a crucial factor in managing fibromyalgia.

Usual dosage level: For rheumatic conditions including fibromyalgia, research suggests a maintenance usage of $1\frac{1}{2}$ dropperfuls of high-quality 100% goji berry extract, two to three times per day at mealtime. During flare-ups, the serving size may be doubled.

CHAPTER 21

HEART (CARDIOVASCULAR) DISEASE

When most people consider heart disease, they tend to think specifically of coronary artery disease, a narrowing of the arteries leading to the heart. It's no wonder—coronary artery disease is the single largest killer of American adults, causing roughly 1.5 million heart attacks each year (about one every 26 seconds).

And yet, as deadly as coronary artery disease may be, it is just one of a number of serious conditions known collectively as cardiovascular disease (CVD)—the number one cause of mortality worldwide with, according to the World Health Organization, 17 million people around the globe dying of cardiovascular disease each year. CVD includes dysfunctional conditions of the heart, arteries and veins that supply oxygen to vital life-sustaining areas of the body like the brain, the heart itself and other vital organs. A lack of oxygen causes the tissue or organ to die.

CVD covers several conditions, including: ischemic heart disease (and stroke), which occurs when blood vessels are obstructed due to excess deposits of cholesterol-laden fat (arteriosclerosis) or plaque (atherosclerosis), which restricts oxygen flow and can result in heart attack or stroke depending on where in the body the obstruction occurs; uncontrolled high blood pressure (hypertension), which can lead to stroke, heart attack, heart failure or kidney failure; arrhythmia—an abnormal rhythm or rate of heartbeat caused by a disturbance in the electrical nerve impulses of the heart, which is often due to arteriosclerosis as a result of inadequate blood supply to the heart muscle; and high cholesterol, which becomes dangerous when the 'bad' (LDL) cholesterol oxidizes in the body, resulting in lipid peroxides that adhere to the walls of arteries in the form of atherosclerotic plaques.

There are several risk factors for heart disease; some are controllable through changes in diet, exercise and behavior. Other risk factors are uncontrollable. CVD afflicts more men on a percentage basis, but women are catching up. CVD is now the number one killer of women, responsible for more deaths than the next seven causes combined! Those over 65 also have an increased risk, yet CVD is the number one killer of all adults over 35. Genetics also plays a large part in the risk for CVD. Post-menopausal women no longer have the heart-protective benefit of reproductive hormones. And race can play a role—those of African or Latin descent are more likely to have heart disease than are Caucasians.

That being said, there is still much you can do to reduce your risk of heart disease. Quitting smoking is a must—smokers have more than twice the risk for heart attack as nonsmokers, and are much more likely to die if they suffer a heart attack. In addition, improving cholesterol levels, controlling high blood pressure, eating a heart-healthy diet, maintaining a healthy weight (excess weight strains the heart and can exacerbate several other heart disease risk factors such as diabetes), exercising (people who don't exercise have higher rates of death and heart disease when compared to those who engage in even gentle activities like walking or gardening), controlling diabetes (if not properly controlled, diabetes can lead to significant heart damage, including heart attacks and death), and managing stress can all lower your risk.

Goji has also been shown to have tremendous benefits when it comes to the prevention of heart disease. First of all, it fights lipid peroxidation in two ways. The accumulation of lipid peroxides in the blood can lead to cardiovascular disease, heart attack, atherosclerosis and stroke. Our blood contains the antioxidant enzyme superoxide dismutase (SOD) to fight against lipid peroxidation, but levels of SOD decrease as we age. In a Ningxia Medical University study, goji berry consumption was accompanied by a remarkable 40 percent increase in SOD levels, and a decrease in lipid peroxides of an impressive 65 percent. It has been noted that goji actually contains a unique iron-containing form of SOD. An investigation by Huang Y et al (1999) in China found that lipid peroxidation was also significantly inhibited by goji's flavonoids. Next, the effects of goji's master molecule polysaccharides on endothelial function were observed by Jia YX et al (1998) in China. Their results showed that the increase of blood pressure in hypertensive rats could be prevented significantly by treatment with goji polysaccharides. And, of course, goji has been known as the secret to weight loss for centuries in Asia (see the Obesity chapter for more details).

Usual dosage level: For all cardiovascular conditions, research suggests a usage of six to twelve sprays, or $1^1/_2$ dropperfuls, twice daily of high-quality 100% goji berry extract, or as directed by a health practitioner.

CHAPTER 22

IMMUNE ENHANCEMENT

Your immune system is designed to attack, neutralize and eliminate substances that don't belong in a healthy body: A strong and smooth-running immune system is your most powerful frontline defense against viruses, bacteria, carcinogens and a host of other toxic or harmful threats to health.

Unfortunately, modern life presents many challenges to proper immune function: aging diminishes immune response; high stress causes elevated levels of the immune-depressing hormone cortisol; inadequate rest or exercise depletes immune reserves; poor nutrition deprives the immune system of essential nutrients; and environmental irritants and airborne pollutants are ever-present.

At the heart of the immune response is the ability to distinguish between your own cells ("self") and foreign invaders ("non-self"). Normally your immune cells do not attack your own body tissues. That is because every cell in your body is encoded on its surface with a pattern of special proteins called the major histocompatibility complex (MHC). Every cell in your body bears the same MHC code, which is also called your "tissue type." There are more than 200 different tissue types, and, like blood type, they are not intercompatible. (That is why doctors must pair organ recipients with donors whose MHC sets match as closely as possible for successful organ transplantations. Otherwise, the recipient's immune system will likely attack the transplant, leading to graft rejection.)

Your immune cells act as security guards, constantly checking the MHC credentials of every cell they encounter. If the code is incorrect, the cell is determined to be non-self and an immune response is triggered. Any non-self substance capable of triggering an immune response is known as an antigen. An antigen can be a whole non-self cell, a bacterium, a virus or even a portion of a protein from a foreign organism.

The organs of your immune system are positioned strategically throughout your body and include bone marrow, the thymus gland and the spleen. These organs produce the immune cells that patrol your body. The organs of your immune system are connected with one another and with other organs of the body by a network of lymphatic vessels, which closely parallel the body's veins and arteries. Cells and fluids are exchanged between blood and lymphatic vessels, enabling the lymphatic system to monitor the body for invading microbes. The lymphatic vessels carry lymph, a clear fluid that bathes the body's tissues.

Cells destined to become immune cells arise in your body's bone marrow from stem cells. There are two main divisions of immune cells—the early-responding and non-specific myeloid cells (which include neutrophils—the first responders, which race to the scene of infection to assess the situation and send out warning signals; macrophages—cells that roam the bloodstream looking for foreign invaders and infected cells, which they surround and gobble up; cytokines—special "messenger proteins" that are produced by the macrophages and speed throughout the body recruiting more macrophages and other immune cells, drawing them to where they are needed; eosinophils—cells that attack parasites by spraying them with killer chemicals; and basophils—cells that release granules containing histamine and other allergy-related molecules) and the later-acting, more targeted lymphocytes (B-cells that originate in the bone marrow and produce antibodies to the invading organism; T-cells—specialized lymphocytes that originate in the thymus gland and act like elite combat commandos to track down and kill viruses and bacteria that are hiding inside body cells and kill tumor cells on contact; and interferons—special proteins that interfere with viruses and neutralize them.)

When your immune system malfunctions, it can unleash a torrent of disorders and diseases:

- **Allergy:** Allergies such as hay fever and hives are related to the antibody known as IgE. The first time an allergy-prone person is exposed to an allergen—for instance, grass pollen—the individual's B-cells make large amounts of grass pollen IgE antibody.
These IgE molecules attach to granule-containing cells known as mast cells, which are plentiful in the lungs, skin, tongue, and linings of the nose and gastrointestinal tract. The next time that person encounters grass pollen, the IgE-primed mast cell releases powerful chemicals that cause the wheezing, sneezing and other symptoms of allergy.

- **Auto-Immune Diseases:** Sometimes the immune system's recognition apparatus breaks down and the body begins to manufacture antibodies and T-cells directed against the body's own cells and organs.

- **AIDS:** When the immune system is lacking one or more of its components, the result is an immunodeficiency disorder. AIDS is caused by a virus that destroys helper T-cells. The virus copies itself incessantly and invades the very cells needed to organize an immune defense. The AIDS virus splices its DNA into the DNA of the cell it infects; the cell is thereafter directed to churn out new viruses.

- **Immunity and Cancer:** When a normal cell becomes cancerous, its surface MHC pattern changes. According to one theory, patrolling cells of the immune system provide continuous body wide surveillance, catching and eliminating cells that undergo malignant transformation. Tumors develop when this immune surveillance breaks down or is overwhelmed.

Fortunately, goji can balance immune response. It is important to note that goji is not an immune booster, as that would be undesirable in cases of autoimmune disorders. As an adaptogen, goji acts as an immune balancer, helping to re-establish normal and healthy immune function. And goji polysaccharides enhance and balance the activity of all classes of immune lymphocyte cells, including T-cells, cytotoxic T-cells, NK cells, lysozyme, inter-leukin-2, tumor necrosis factor-alpha and the immunoglobulins IgG and IgA. Goji not only increases lymphocyte count; it also helps to activate them when the body is under attack.

In Asia, the goji berry has also been used as a primary allergy therapy for centuries. The noted ethnobotanist Dr. James A. Duke classifies goji as an immunomodulator—an enhancing substance that can balance and normalize abnormal immune response.

Goji's antioxidants and unique master molecule polysaccharides also have the ability to restore and repair vital DNA, preventing cancerous genetic mutations that might otherwise overwhelm the immune system. Goji also has the ability to cause the death of tumor cells by inducing apoptosis; a process in which cancer cells are broken down and recycled.

Usual dosage level: For immune enhancement, research and traditional use suggest a daily intake of six to twelve sprays, or $1^1/_2$ dropperfuls, of high-quality 100% goji berry extract.

CHAPTER 23

OBESITY

Nearly two-thirds of Americans aged 20 years and older are overweight. More than three of every ten American adults are significantly overweight—a condition termed obesity. Both overweight and obesity are associated with increased health risk for a host of chronic diseases. In fact, a March 2004 study published in the *Journal of the American Medical Association* cited obesity and its complications as the second leading cause of preventable death.

The problem is not uniquely American. In 1995, a survey by the World Health Organization estimated the global number of obese adults to be 200 million. A mere five years later, the number had jumped incredibly to 300 million. Justifiably alarmed, the organization has given a name to this seemingly unstoppable worldwide epidemic—globesity.

Most people tend to use the terms *overweight* and *obese* interchangeably, but in fact, they have quite different meanings.

Overweight indicates a body weight that exceeds established standards. The excess weight does not necessarily come from fat. If you're a bodybuilder, professional athlete or just someone with "big bones," you may be overweight but not obese.

Obesity refers specifically to those individuals whose excess body weight is a result of a high percentage of body fat. Although experts had long debated the threshold points separating normal weight, overweight and obesity, there is now near-unanimous agreement thanks to the development of a statistical tool known as the body mass index or BMI—a mathematical formula that uses your height and weight to generate a number score that indicates the extent of overweight.

Either of these formulas can be used to determine your BMI:

$$BMI = \text{Weight in pounds} \div$$
$$(\text{Height in inches} \times \text{Height in inches}) \times 703$$

$$BMI = \text{Weight in kilograms} \div$$
$$(\text{Height in meters} \times \text{Height in meters})$$

For adults over 20 years old (who are not pregnant), BMI falls into one of these categories:

Below 18.5	Underweight
18.5–24.9	Normal
25.0–29.9	Overweight
30.0 and above	Obese

In scientific terms, obesity occurs when you consume more calories than you burn. What causes this imbalance between calories in and calories out may differ from one person to another. Genetic, environmental, psychological and other factors may all play a part. Perhaps the most important cause of obesity is something that we all face—the everyday stress of modern life. When under chronic stress, your adrenal glands overproduce the hormone cortisol. Although cortisol is necessary in normal amounts, an excess of this stress hormone can create a cascade of harmful side effects, many of which can cause weight gain, including: activation of fat-storage hormones and enzymes; conversion of protein in the body into unwanted sugar and fat; halt in secretion of fat-burning human growth hormone (hGH); accumulation of dangerous "apple-type" abdominal fat; increase in appetite and cravings for sweet and fatty foods; and progressive insulin resistance, which leads to type 2 diabetes, hypertension, cardiovascular disease and the other health risks associated with obesity.

Researchers at UCLA and elsewhere have demonstrated conclusively the interconnection between stress and high cortisol levels. If you can reduce stress, you will minimize or eliminate the harmful effects of cortisol.

For more than a thousand years, traditional Asian medicine has been successfully addressing the problem by the use of adaptogens. The term refers to certain herbs that help the body to adapt to stress. No adaptogenic herb is more renowned than the goji berry for reducing mental and emotional stress. It has been suggested that goji's unique stress-lowering ability can help to normalize cortisol levels. If you can end the cortisol cascade, you'll soon be on your way to a lower body mass index and a healthier weight. You'll also notice an impressive array of benefits for whole body good health, including: increased fat burning; less fat storage; reduction of food cravings; more energy; less fatigue after eating; and much more.

In addition, an Asian anti-obesity study showed that patients who were given goji each morning and each afternoon had excellent results, with most patients losing significant weight. And in an animal study, it was shown that goji's master molecule polysaccharides enhanced the conversion of food into energy and reduced body weight.

Usual dosage level: For weight management, research suggests a daily intake of six sprays, or $1\frac{1}{2}$ dropperfuls, of high-quality 100% goji berry extract before each meal. If you are a night eater, add six sprays at 8:00 pm.

CHAPTER 24

SEXUAL DYSFUNCTION

If you watch prime-time TV dramas or listen to lyrics of current pop songs, you might think that sex is only for younger adults. This simply isn't true. Sexual feelings and desires are with us throughout our entire lives. In fact, according to the Mayo Foundation for Medical Research and Education, most people still have sexual fantasies and desires well into their eighties and nineties.

Although sex in your middle or later years may be a bit different from the way it was in your twenties, it can be every bit as enjoyable and fulfilling. All that's required is an understanding of the normal changes that are taking place in your body and your partner's body. These changes can affect your ability to have and enjoy sex and, if not addressed, they can result in difficulties with arousal or performance (sexual dysfunction).

Your libido (sex drive) is regulated by the hormone testosterone. Although classified as a male hormone, testosterone is produced by both men and women. As you age, your body produces less testosterone. The result? Your interest in sex may diminish significantly.

Men and women experience different changes in their bodies as they age. As women approach menopause, they experience a drop in levels of the female hormones estrogen and progesterone, which can make sexual activity uncomfortable or even painful. Changing hormone levels can also cause sleeping problems and can result in heavy, irregular or lengthy menstrual periods. As men get older, erectile dysfunction (ED) becomes more common. Also referred to as impotence, ED is the loss of ability to have and sustain an erection firm enough for sexual intercourse. According to the National Institute on Aging, by age 65 about 15 to 25 percent of men have this problem at least one out of every four times they are having sex. This may happen in men with heart disease, high blood pressure or diabetes—either because of the disease or the medicines used to treat it.

Freedom from stress and distraction are required elements for arousal and sexual performance. For men, if you are overly stressed with worries about how you will perform, it can trigger impotence. Ample reserves of stamina and endurance are also necessary for a stress-free sexual experience. In addition, various age-related diseases can affect your sexual performance, or passion. Joint pain from arthritis can make sexual contact uncomfortable. Exercise, rest, warm baths and changing the position or timing of sexual activity can be helpful. Diabetes is one of the few illnesses that can cause impotence in men, and heart disease (narrowing and hardening of the arteries, known as atherosclerosis, can change blood vessels so that blood does not flow freely) can lead to trouble with erections in men as can high blood pressure.

Fortunately, goji can help with all of the aforementioned conditions (see particular chapters for details), and you can revive your sex drive with goji. Goji berries have been traditionally regarded in Asia as a longevity, strength-building and sexual potency food of the highest order. In several study groups with elderly people, the berry was given once a day for three weeks. The results showed that spirit and optimism increased significantly in all patients. Additionally, nearly all patients reported improved appetite and better quality of sleep. More than 35 percent of the patients saw a marked recovery of sexual function.

The noted herbalist Ron Teeguarden reports that, in Chinese studies, goji was shown to markedly increase testosterone levels in the blood, increasing libido in test subjects.

And goji boosts stamina. An animal study showed that goji's master molecule polysaccharides induced a remarkable increase in exercise tolerance and stamina and helped to eliminate fatigue.

When taken orally, it markedly increases androgen levels in the blood, making patients feel more energetic.

So potent is the goji berry that an ancient Chinese proverb cautions men who are traveling far from their wives and families as follows: "He who travels one thousand kilometers from home should not eat goji!"

Usual dosage level: Research and traditional use suggest a daily intake of $1^1/_2$ dropperfuls, of high-quality 100% goji berry extract, taken with meals. It can also be taken before sex.

CONCLUSION

I have endeavored in these pages to impart to the reader a measure of my profound respect and admiration for the remarkable goji. I owe an immeasurable debt of gratitude to the generations of Himalayan healers who, through the ages, have protected, cherished and preserved this unique gift of Nature.

Now, it is your turn. My fondest wish is that you will honor the Himalayan tradition and share your newly found enlightenment with everyone whom you love and cherish.

As the ancient poet wisely counseled, *"Drink . . . and enjoy a long life."* And when you do, please remember to raise your glass to the Himalayans for sharing with the world their secret for health and long life!

ADDITIONAL RESEARCH-SUPPORTED USES OF GOJI

Blood Builder

Usual dosage level: $1^1/_2$ dropperfuls daily

A study in China showed LBP facilitated stem cell proliferation and increased the number of monocytes in bone marrow. LBP helps the monocytes to convert to matured leukocytes.

The berry has also been used in a number of recent clinical trials for treatment of bone marrow deficiency conditions (low production of red blood cells, white blood cells, and platelets).

Another three-year clinical study investigated the effects of the goji berry on the immune, physiological and biochemical indexes of the blood of aged volunteers. The results indicated that the goji berry caused the blood of older people to revert to a markedly younger state.

Energy

Usual dosage level: $1^1/_2$ dropperfuls three times daily

An animal study showed that goji's LBP polysaccharides induced a remarkable increase in exercise tolerance and stamina, and helped to eliminate fatigue. Goji LBP enhances glycogen storage (glycogen is the body's primary energy fuel).

Hypertension (high blood pressure)

Usual dosage level: $1^1/_2$ dropperfuls twice daily

The effects of *Lycium barbarum* polysaccharides (LBP) on endothelial function were observed by Jia YX et al (1998) in China. Their results showed that the increase of blood pressure in hypertensive rats could be prevented significantly by treatment with goji LBP.

Infertility

Usual dosage level: $1^1/_2$ dropperfuls three times daily

Goji berries have long been used by Asian physicians for the treatment of infertility. However, the active ingredients and the mechanism of action remain unknown. Wang Y et al (2002) tried to explore this area by studying the effect of goji polysaccharides (LBP) on cultured sperm epithelial cells. They reported that LBP inhibited hyperthermia-induced structural damage in murine seminiferous epithelium, in vitro. They also found that the goji polysaccharides extended the life of the cells.

Oxidative stress was reported to be a major cause of structural degradation and cell death in testicular cells. Wang Y et al (2002) assayed the effect of LBP on ultra-violet (UV) light-induced lipid peroxidation and cytochrome c reduction by free radicals. They found that the polysaccharides of goji berry were potent inhibitors of both reactions. Their results demonstrated the antioxidant mechanism of action for the protective effect of LBP and provided a scientific basis for the traditional use of goji berry for treatment of infertility.

Liver Protection

Usual dosage level: $1^1/_2$ dropperfuls daily

A new cerebroside was isolated from the goji berry that could protect the liver cells of rats from the toxicity induced by carbon tetrachloride. In a further study, Kim SY et al (1999) postulated that the *Lycium* cerebrosides may preserve hepatic mitochondrial levels of glutathione by scavenging reactive oxygen species produced and thereby reduce lipid peroxidation and cellular damage.

Periodontal Disease

Usual dosage level: $1^1/_2$ dropperfuls two times daily

The effects of goji on attachment and growth of human gingival fibroblasts to root surfaces *in vitro* were investigated by Liu B (1992) at Fourth Military Medical University in Xian, China. His results revealed that LBP (goji polysaccharides), even at low doses, could improve attachment and growth of fibroblast on the planed diseased root surfaces to a certain extent. His results suggested that goji may improve the formation of new attachment of periodontal tissue.

Vision Improvement

Usual dosage level: $1^1/_2$ dropperfuls twice daily

Goji berries were very popular for their vision improvement properties in ancient China. Modern Chinese scientists found goji berries able to reduce dark adapting time and improve vision under subdued light.

Physiologic scotoma (blind spots) decreased and vitamin A increased in patients after taking goji berries.

BIBLIOGRAPHY

Agrawal, D.P. and J.S. Kharakwal. 1998. *Central Himalayas: an Archaeological, Linguistic and Culural Synthesis*. New Delhi: Aryan Books International.

Agrawal, D.P., D.S. Pokharia, A.N. Upreti. 1997. Central Himalayan Folklore (*Jagars*) in an Inter-Disciplinary Perspective, (ed.) Khanduri B. M. & Nautiyal Vinod, *Him Kanti: Archaeology, Art and History*. Delhi: Book India Publishing Company, pp. 173–183.

Arias, E. United States Life Tables, 2000–2002. National Center for Health Statistics. National Vital Statistics Reports; Vol. 51 No. 3. Hyattsville, MD. Hyun M, Jakes S, Kite H, Oda Y, McGirk T. "Long Lives Well Lived." *TIME Asia*, 21 July 2003, 162.

Cao GW, Yang WG, Du P. 1994. *Observation of the Effects of LAK/IL-2 Therapy Combined with Lycium Barbarum Polysaccharides in the Treatment of 75 Cancer Patients.* Chunghua Chung Liu Tsa Chih. 1994 Nov, 16(6): 428–431.

Cole, S. 2000. The Myth of Fingerprints: A forensic science stands trial. *Lingua Franca* 2000 Vol. 10 No. 8, pp. 54–62.

Dharmananda, S. 1997. *Lycium Fruit*. Institute for Traditional Medicine, Portland, Oregon. ONLINE. Available: www.aloe-info.nl/lycium.htm [29 July 2003].

Ding Aurong, Li Shuli. 1990. *Effects on Activities of Na+, K+-ATP Enzymes from Huang Jing and Five Other Herbs.* Zhong Cheng Yao (Chinese Patent Herbs). 1990, (9): 28.

Gan L, Wang J, Zhang S. 2001. *Inhibition the growth of human leukemia cells by Lycium barbarum polysaccharide*. Wei Sheng Yan Jiu. 2001 Nov, 30(6): 333–5.

Geng Changshan, Wang Geying, Lin Yongdong, et al.1988. *Effects on Mouse Lymphocyte and T Cells from Lycium Barbarum Polysaccharide (LBP).* Zhong Cao Yao (Chinese Herbs). 1988, 19(7): 25.

He Jie, Pan Li, Guo Fuxiang, et al. 1993. *Hepatoprotective Effects from Lycium Barbarum Fruit in a Mouse Experiment.* China Pharmacology and Toxicology. 1993, 7(4): 293.

Huang Guifang, Luo Jieying. 1990. *Immune Boosting Effects from Fu Fang Wu Zi Yang Zong Wan (a Chinese patent herb containing Lycium barbarum fruit).* Zhong Cao Yao (Chinese Herbs). 1990, 12(6): 27.

Huang Y et al. 1999. *The protective effects of total flavonoids from Lycium barbarum L. on lipid peroxidation of liver mitochondria and red blood cell in rats.* Wei Sheng Yan Jiu. 28: 115–6.

Jia YX, Dong JW, Wu XX, Ma TM, Shi AY. 1998. *The effect of Lycium barbarum polysaccharide on vascular tension in two-kidney, one clip model of hypertension.* Sheng Li Xue Bao. 1998 Jun, 50(3): 309–14.

Kim HP, Kim SY, Lee EJ, Kim YC. 1997. *Zeaxanthin Dipalmitate from Lycium Barbarum Has Hepatoprotective Activity.* Res. Commun Mol Pathol Pharmacol. 1997 Sep, (3): 301–314.

Kinsella, K., Velkoff, V. 2001. *An Aging World: 2001.* U.S. Census Bureau, Series P95/01–1, U.S. Government Printing Office, Washington, DC.

Kious, WJ, Tilling, R. *This Dynamic Earth: The Story of Plate Tectonics.* ONLINE. 1996. US Geological Survey. Available: http: //pubs.usgs.gov/publications/text/ himalaya.html. [19 July 2003].

Levy, T. 2002. *Vitamin C, Infectious Diseases, and Toxins: Curing the Incurable.* Philadelphia, PA: Xlibris Corporation, pp. 33–38.

Li Wei, Dai Shouzhi, Ma Fu, et al. 1991. *Active Lymphocyte Effects Observed after Taking Lycium Barbarum Fruits.* Zhong Cao Yao (Chinese Herbs). 1991, 22(6): 251.

Li yuhao, Deng Xiangchao, Wu Heqing, et al. 1994. *The Effect on Lipid Metabolism of Injured Liver Cells in Rat.* Zhong Guo Zhong Yao Za Zhi (Journal of Chinese Herbal Medicine). 1994, 19(5): 300.

Liu B. 1992. *Effect of Lycium barbarum L and Drynaria fortunei J Smith on in vitro attachment and growth of human gingival fibroblasts on root surfaces.* Zhonghua Kou Qiang Yi Xue Za Zhi. 27: 159–61.

Lu CX, Cheng BQ. 1991. *Radiosensitizing Effects of Lycium Barbarum Polysaccharide of Lewis Lung Cancer.* Chung His I chieh Ho Tsa Chih. 1991, Oct: 11(10): 611–612.

Luo Q, Yan J, Zhang S. 2000. *Isolation and purification of Lycium barbarum polysaccharides and its antifatigue effect.* Wei Sheng Yan Jiu. 2000 Mar 30, 29(2): 115–7.

Marquess Cuzon of Kedleston. 1984. *"A Viceroy's India" Leaves from Lord Curzon's Notebook.* Sidgwick & Jackson. London, England.

Pastor, PN, Makuc, DM, Reuben, C, Xia, H. 2002. *Health, United States, 2002 with Chartbook on Trends in the Health of Americans.* National Center for Health Statistics, Hyattsville, MD.

Qi L, Zhou, R, Wang, Y, Zhu, Y. 1998. *Study on Reducing Monosaccharides of Lycium Barbarum Separation in Capillary Zone Electrophoresis.* Beijing institute of New Technology Application. Beijing, China. Published in *Proceedings of the Second Asia-Pacific International Symposium on Capillary Electrophoresis and related Microscale Techniques (APCE98)*.

Qi Zongshao, Li Shufang, Wu Jiping, et al. 1986. *Chemical Analysis on Lycium Barbarum Fruit and Leaves*. Zhong Yao Tong Bao (Chinese Herb News). 1986, 11(3): 41.

Salvemini D, Riley D, Cuzzocrea S. 2002. *Review: SOD Mimetics are Coming of Age*. Nature Reviews Drug Discovery. 2002 May, 1(5): 367–374.

Schomberg, Reginald Charles Francis. 1936. *Between the Oxus and the Indus*. London: Martin Hopkinson. [Reprint Lahore: Al-Biruni 1976].

Tao Maoxuan, Zhao Zhongliang. 1992. *In Vitro Anti-Mutation Effect of Lycium Barbarum Polysaccharide (LBP)*. Zong Cao Yao (Chinese Herbs). 1992, 23(9): 474.

Teeguarden, R. 2000. *The Ancient Wisdom of the Chinese Tonic Herbs*. Warner Books.

Teeguarden, R. 2002. *Quality Chinese Herbs. Lycium Fruit*. ONLINE. Available: www.qualitychineseherbs.com/herbal_ingredients/lycium_fruit.htm [22 July 2003].

The Tanaduk International Botanical Research Institute. 2003. *Tanaduk Institute Initiates New Studies with Tibetan Berries*. Monograph 91 (CIR/R) - Research Study. The Tanaduk International Botanical Research Institute, Eastsound, WA.

Tiwari, L. *Traditional Himalayan Medicine System and Its Materia Medica*. ONLINE. 2003. The Infinity Foundation. Available: www.infinityfoundation.com/mandala/t_es/t_es_tiwar_medica.htm. [29 June 2003].

Travel Himalayas. *Himalayas: The Legendary Majestic Beauty*. ONLINE. Available: www.travel-himalayas.com/about-himalayas [20 July 2003] Visit Himalaya. *Himalaya —A Dream for All Explorers*. ONLINE. Available: http://wvvw.visithimalaya.com [27 July 2003].

Wang Qiang, Chen Suiqing, Zhang Zhehua, et al. 1991. *The Measurement of Lycium Barbarum Polysaccharide (LBP) in Lycium Barbarum Fruit*. Zhong Cao Yao (Chinese Herbs). 1991, 22(2): 67.

Wang Y et al. 2002. *Protective effect of Fructus Lycii polysaccharides against time and hyperthermia-induced damage in cultured seminiferous epithelium*. J.Ethnopharmacol 82: 169.

Wrench, GT. 1938. *The Wheel of Health: a study of a very healthy people*. The C. W. Daniel Company Ltd., London, England.

Zhang M, Wang J, Zhang S. 2002. *Study on the composition of Lycium barbarum polysaccharides and its effects on the growth of weanling mice*. Wei Sheng Yan Jiu. 2002 Apr, 31(2): 118–9.

Zhang X. 1993. *Experimental research on the role of Lycium barbarum polysaccharide in anti-peroxidation*. Zhongguo Zhong Yao Za Zhi. 18: 110–2, pg. 38.

RESEARCH PAPERS
ON LYCIUM BARBARUM

Lycium Barbarum Human

Adams M, Wiedenmann M, Tittel G, Bauer R. HPLC-MS trace analysis of atropine in Lycium barbarum berries. *Phytochem Anal.* 2006 Sep; 17(5): 279–83.

Amagase H, Nance DM. A randomized, double-blind, placebo-controlled, clinical study of the general effects of a standardized Lycium barbarum (Goji) Juice, GoChi. *J Altern Complement Med.* 2008 May; 14(4): 403–12.

Amagase H, Nance DM. Lycium barbarum increases caloric expenditure and decreases waist circumference in healthy overweight men and women: pilot study. *J Am Coll Nutr.* 2011 Oct; 30(5): 304–9.

Amagase H, Sun B, Borek C. Lycium barbarum (goji) juice improves in vivo antioxidant biomarkers in serum of healthy adults. *Nutr Res.* 2009 Jan; 29(1): 19–25.

Amagase H, Sun B, Nance DM. Immunomodulatory effects of a standardized Lycium barbarum fruit juice in Chinese older healthy human subjects. *J Med Food.* 2009 Oct; 12(5): 1159–65.

Arroyo-Martinez Q, Sáenz MJ, Argüelles Arias F, Acosta MS. Lycium barbarum: a new hepatotoxic "natural" agent? *Dig Liver Dis.* 2011 Sep; 43(9): 749. Epub 2011 May 31. No abstract available.

Benzie IF, Chung WY, Wang J, Richelle M, Bucheli P. Enhanced bioavailability of zeaxanthin in a milk-based formulation of wolfberry (Gou Qi Zi; Fructus barbarum L.). *Br J Nutr.* 2006 Jul; 96(1): 154–60.

Breithaupt DE, Weller P, Wolters M, Hahn A. Comparison of plasma responses in human subjects after the ingestion of 3R,3R'-zeaxanthin dipalmitate from wolfberry (Lycium barbarum) and non-esterified 3R,3R'-zeaxanthin using chiral high-performance liquid chromatography. *Br J Nutr.* 2004 May; 91(5): 707–13.

Bucheli P, Vidal K, Shen L, Gu Z, Zhang C, Miller LE, Wang J. Goji berry effects on macular characteristics and plasma antioxidant levels. *Optom Vis Sci.* 2011 Feb; 88(2): 257–62.

Cassileth B. Lycium (Lycium barbarum). *Oncology* (Williston Park). 2010 Dec; 24(14): 1353.

Chang RC, So KF. Use of anti-aging herbal medicine, Lycium barbarum, against aging-associated diseases. What do we know so far? *Cell Mol Neurobiol.* 2008 Aug; 28(5): 643–52. Epub 2007 Aug 21. Review.

Chao JC, Chiang SW, Wang CC, Tsai YH, Wu MS. Hot water-extracted Lycium barbarum and Rehmannia glutinosa inhibit proliferation and induce apoptosis of hepatocellular carcinoma cells. *World J Gastroenterol.* 2006 Jul 28; 12(28): 4478–84.

Cheng CY, Chung WY, Szeto YT, Benzie IF. Fasting plasma zeaxanthin response to Fructus barbarum L. (wolfberry; Kei Tze) in a food-based human supplementation trial. *Br J Nutr.* 2005 Jan; 93(1): 123–30.

Gan L, Zhang SH, Liu Q, Xu HB. A polysaccharide-protein complex from Lycium barbarum upregulates cytokine expression in human peripheral blood mononuclear cells. *Eur J Pharmacol.* 2003 Jun 27; 471(3): 217–22.

Gong H, Shen P, Jin L, Xing C, Tang F. Therapeutic effects of Lycium barbarum polysaccharide (LBP) on irradiation or chemotherapy-induced myelosuppressive mice. *Cancer Biother Radiopharm.* 2005 Apr; 20(2): 155–62.

Ji J, Wang G, Wang J, Wang P. Functional analysis of multiple carotenogenic genes from Lycium barbarum and Gentiana lutea L. for their effects on beta-carotene production in transgenic tobacco. *Biotechnol Lett.* 2009 Feb; 31(2): 305–12. Epub 2008 Oct 21.

Lam AY, Elmer GW, Mohutsky MA. Possible interaction between warfarin and Lycium barbarum L. *Ann Pharmacother.* 2001 Oct; 35(10): 1199–201.

Leung H, Hung A, Hui AC, Chan TY. Warfarin overdose due to the possible effects of Lycium barbarum L. *Food Chem Toxicol.* 2008 May; 46(5): 1860–2. Epub 2008 Jan 15.

Li G, Sepkovic DW, Bradlow HL, Telang NT, Wong GY. Lycium barbarum inhibits growth of estrogen receptor positive human breast cancer cells by favorably altering estradiol metabolism. *Nutr Cancer.* 2009; 61(3): 408–14.

Lin NC, Lin JC, Chen SH, Ho CT, Yeh AI. Effect of Goji (Lycium barbarum) on expression of genes related to cell survival. *J Agric Food Chem.* 2011 Sep 28; 59(18): 10088–96. Epub 2011 Aug 25.

Luo Q, Li Z, Yan J, Zhu F, Xu RJ, Cai YZ. Lycium barbarum polysaccharides induce apoptosis in human prostate cancer cells and inhibits prostate cancer growth in a xenograft mouse model of human prostate cancer. *J Med Food.* 2009 Aug; 12(4): 695–703.

Lycium barbarum. *J Soc Integr Oncol.* 2007 Summer; 5(3): 130. No abstract available.

Mao F, Xiao B, Jiang Z, Zhao J, Huang X, Guo J. Anticancer effect of Lycium barbarum polysaccharides on colon cancer cells involves G0/G1 phase arrest. *Med Oncol.* 2011 Mar; 28(1): 121–6. Epub 2010 Jan 12.

Miao Y, Xiao B, Jiang Z, Guo Y, Mao F, Zhao J, Huang X, Guo J. Growth inhibition and cell-cycle arrest of human gastric cancer cells by Lycium barbarum polysaccharide. *Med Oncol.* 2010 Sep; 27(3): 785–90. Epub 2009 Aug 11.

Monzón Ballarín S, López-Matas MA, Sáenz Abad D, Pérez-Cinto N, Carnés J. Anaphylaxis associated with the ingestion of Goji berries (Lycium barbarum). *J Investig Allergol Clin Immunol.* 2011; 21(7): 567–70.

Potterat O. Goji (Lycium barbarum and L. chinense): Phytochemistry, pharmacology and safety in the perspective of traditional uses and recent popularity. *Planta Med.* 2010 Jan; 76(1): 7–19. Epub 2009 Oct 20. Review.

Reeve VE, Allanson M, Arun SJ, Domanski D, Painter N. Mice drinking goji berry juice (Lycium barbarum) are protected from UV radiation-induced skin damage via antioxidant pathways. *Photochem Photobiol Sci.* 2010 Apr; 9(4): 601–7.

Seeram NP. Berry fruits: compositional elements, biochemical activities, and the impact of their intake on human health, performance, and disease. *J Agric Food Chem.* 2008 Feb 13; 56(3): 627–9. Epub 2008 Jan 23.

Song MK, Roufogalis BD, Huang TH. Reversal of the Caspase-Dependent Apoptotic Cytotoxicity Pathway by Taurine from Lycium barbarum (Goji Berry) in Human Retinal Pigment Epithelial Cells: Potential Benefit in Diabetic Retinopathy. *Evid Based Complement Alternat Med.* 2012; 2012: 323784. Epub 2012 Apr 11.

Song MK, Salam NK, Roufogalis BD, Huang TH. Lycium barbarum (Goji Berry) extracts and its taurine component inhibit PPAR-γ-dependent gene transcription in human retinal pigment epithelial cells: Possible implications for diabetic retinopathy treatment. *Biochem Pharmacol.* 2011 Nov 1; 82(9): 1209–18. Epub 2011 Jul 27.

Vidal K, Bucheli P, Gao Q, Moulin J, Shen LS, Wang J, Blum S, Benyacoub J. Immunomodulatory effects of dietary supplementation with a milk-based wolfberry formulation in healthy elderly: a randomized, double-blind, placebo-controlled trial. *Rejuvenation Res.* 2012 Feb; 15(1): 89–97.

Wang XY, Wang YG, Wang YF. Ginsenoside Rb1, Rg1 and three extracts of traditional Chinese medicine attenuate ultraviolet B-induced G1 growth arrest in HaCaT cells and dermal fibroblasts involve down-regulating the expression of p16, p21 and p53. *Photodermatol Photoimmunol Photomed.* 2011 Aug; 27(4): 203–12. doi: 10.1111/j.1600-0781.2011.00601.x.

Wu PS, Wu SJ, Tsai YH, Lin YH, Chao JC. Hot water extracted Lycium barbarum and Rehmannia glutinosa inhibit liver inflammation and fibrosis in rats. *Am J Chin Med.* 2011; 39(6): 1173–91.

Wu WB, Hung DK, Chang FW, Ong ET, Chen BH. Anti-inflammatory and anti-angiogenic effects of flavonoids isolated from Lycium barbarum Linnaeus on human umbilical vein endothelial cells. *Food Funct.* 2012 Jul 3. [Epub ahead of print]

Xin YF, Zhou GL, Deng ZY, Chen YX, Wu YG, Xu PS, Xuan YX. Protective effect of Lycium barbarum on doxorubicin-induced cardiotoxicity. *Phytother Res.* 2007 Nov; 21(11): 1020–4.

Yang RM, Suo YR, Wang HL. [Determination and analysis of trace elements in Lycium barbarum L. from different regions of Qinghai province]. *Guang Pu Xue Yu Guang Pu Fen Xi.* 2012 Feb; 32(2): 525–8. Chinese.

Zhang M, Chen H, Huang J, Li Z, Zhu C, Zhang S. Effect of lycium barbarum polysaccharide on human hepatoma QGY7703 cells: inhibition of proliferation and induction of apoptosis. *Life Sci.* 2005 Mar 18; 76(18): 2115-24.

Zhang Z, Liu X, Wu T, Liu J, Zhang X, Yang X, Goodheart MJ, Engelhardt JF, Wang Y. Selective suppression of cervical cancer Hela cells by 2-O-β-D-glucopyranosyl-L-ascorbic acid isolated from the fruit of Lycium barbarum L. *Cell Biol Toxicol.* 2011 Apr; 27(2): 107-21. Epub 2010 Aug 19.

Zhao H, Alexeev A, Chang E, Greenburg G, Bojanowski K. Lycium barbarum glycoconjugates: effect on human skin and cultured dermal fibroblasts. *Phytomedicine.* 2005 Jan; 12(1-2): 131-7.

Zhu CP, Zhang SH. Lycium barbarum polysaccharide inhibits the proliferation of HeLa cells by inducing apoptosis. *J Sci Food Agric.* 2012 Jun 13. doi: 10.1002/jsfa.5743. [Epub ahead of print]

Lycium Barbarum Clinical

Amagase H, Nance DM. A randomized, double-blind, placebo-controlled, clinical study of the general effects of a standardized Lycium barbarum (Goji) Juice, GoChi. *J Altern Complement Med.* 2008 May; 14(4): 403-12.

Amagase H, Nance DM. Lycium barbarum increases caloric expenditure and decreases waist circumference in healthy overweight men and women: pilot study. *J Am Coll Nutr.* 2011 Oct; 30(5): 304-9.

Amagase H, Sun B, Borek C. Lycium barbarum (goji) juice improves in vivo antioxidant biomarkers in serum of healthy adults. *Nutr Res.* 2009 Jan; 29(1): 19-25.

Amagase H, Sun B, Nance DM. Immunomodulatory effects of a standardized Lycium barbarum fruit juice in Chinese older healthy human subjects. *J Med Food.* 2009 Oct; 12(5): 1159-65.

Breithaupt DE, Weller P, Wolters M, Hahn A. Comparison of plasma responses in human subjects after the ingestion of 3R,3R'-zeaxanthin dipalmitate from wolfberry (Lycium barbarum) and non-esterified 3R,3R'-zeaxanthin using chiral high-performance liquid chromatography. *Br J Nutr.* 2004 May; 91(5): 707-13.

Chen Z, Lu J, Srinivasan N, Tan BK, Chan SH. Polysaccharide-protein complex from Lycium barbarum L. is a novel stimulus of dendritic cell immunogenicity. *J Immunol.* 2009 Mar 15; 182(6): 3503-9.

Cheng CY, Chung WY, Szeto YT, Benzie IF. Fasting plasma zeaxanthin response to Fructus barbarum L. (wolfberry; Kei Tze) in a food-based human supplementation trial. *Br J Nutr.* 2005 Jan; 93(1): 123-30.

Ho YS, Yu MS, Yang XF, So KF, Yuen WH, Chang RC. Neuroprotective effects of polysaccharides from wolfberry, the fruits of Lycium barbarum, against homocysteine-induced toxicity in rat cortical neurons. *J Alzheimers Dis.* 2010; 19(3): 813-27.

Potterat O. Goji (Lycium barbarum and L. chinense): Phytochemistry, pharmacology and safety in the perspective of traditional uses and recent popularity. *Planta Med.* 2010 Jan; 76(1): 7-19. Epub 2009 Oct 20. Review.

Vidal K, Bucheli P, Gao Q, Moulin J, Shen LS, Wang J, Blum S, Benyacoub J. Immunomodulatory effects of dietary supplementation with a milk-based wolfberry formulation in healthy elderly: a randomized, double-blind, placebo-controlled trial. *Rejuvenation Res.* 2012 Feb; 15(1): 89–97.

Xin Y, Zhang S, Gu L, Liu S, Gao H, You Z, Zhou G, Wen L, Yu J, Xuan Y. Electro-cardiographic and biochemical evidence for the cardioprotective effect of antioxidants in acute doxorubicin-induced cardiotoxicity in the beagle dogs. *Biol Pharm Bull.* 2011; 34(10): 1523–6.

Goji Antioxidants

Amagase H, Sun B, Borek C. Lycium barbarum (goji) juice improves in vivo antioxidant biomarkers in serum of healthy adults. *Nutr Res.* 2009 Jan; 29(1): 19–25.

Are some of the more exotic berry types, such as goji and açaí berries, better for health than the more common berries such as strawberries, blueberries and raspberries? *Mayo Clin Health Lett.* 2010 Nov; 28(11): 8. No abstract available.

Bucheli P, Vidal K, Shen L, Gu Z, Zhang C, Miller LE, Wang J. Goji berry effects on macular characteristics and plasma antioxidant levels. *Optom Vis Sci.* 2011 Feb; 88(2): 257–62.

Farva D, Goji IA, Joseph PK, Augusti KT. Effects of garlic oil on streptozotocin-diabetic rats maintained on normal and high fat diets. *Indian J Biochem Biophys.* 1986 Feb; 23(1): 24–7. No abstract available.

Hasegawa G, Nakano K, Ienaga K. Serum accumulation of a creatinine oxidative metabolite (NZ-419: 5-hydroxy-1- methylhydatoin) as an intrinsic antioxidant in diabetic patients with or without chronic kidney disease. *Clin Nephrol.* 2011 Oct; 76(4): 284–9.

Hasegawa G, Yamamoto Y, Zhi JG, Tanino Y, Yamasaki M, Yano M, Nakajima T, Fukui M, Yoshikawa T, Nakamura N. Daily profile of plasma %CoQ10 level, a biomarker of oxidative stress, in patients with diabetes manifesting postprandial hyperglycaemia. *Acta Diabetol.* 2005 Dec; 42(4): 179–81.

Kodama S, Yagi R, Ninomiya M, Goji K, Takahashi T, Morishita Y, Matsuo T. The effect of a high fat diet on pyruvate decarboxylase deficiency without central nervous system involvement. *Brain Dev.* 1983; 5(4): 381–9.

Lin NC, Lin JC, Chen SH, Ho CT, Yeh AI. Effect of Goji (Lycium barbarum) on expression of genes related to cell survival. *J Agric Food Chem.* 2011 Sep 28; 59(18): 10088–96. Epub 2011 Aug 25.

Navarro P, Nicolas TS, Gabaldon JA, Mercader-Ros MT, Calín-Sánchez A, Carbonell-Barrachina AA, Pérez-López AJ. Effects of cyclodextrin type on vitamin C, antioxidant activity, and sensory attributes of a mandarin juice enriched with pomegranate and goji berries. *J Food Sci.* 2011 Jun–Jul; 76(5): S319–24. doi: 10.1111/j.1750-3841.2011 .02176.x. Epub 2011 Apr 27.

Potterat O. Goji (Lycium barbarum and L. chinense): Phytochemistry, pharmacology and safety in the perspective of traditional uses and recent popularity. *Planta Med.* 2010 Jan; 76(1): 7–19. Epub 2009 Oct 20. Review.

Reeve VE, Allanson M, Arun SJ, Domanski D, Painter N. Mice drinking goji berry juice (Lycium barbarum) are protected from UV radiation-induced skin damage via antioxidant pathways. *Photochem Photobiol Sci.* 2010 Apr; 9(4): 601–7.

Temple NJ. The marketing of dietary supplements in North America: the emperor is (almost) naked. *J Altern Complement Med.* 2010 Jul; 16(7): 803–6.

Zhang Z, Liu X, Zhang X, Liu J, Hao Y, Yang X, Wang Y. Comparative evaluation of the antioxidant effects of the natural vitamin C analog 2-O-β-D-glucopyranosyl-L-ascorbic acid isolated from Goji berry fruit. *Arch Pharm Res.* 2011 May; 34(5): 801–10. Epub 2011 Jun 9.

Lycium Barbarum Goji

Amagase H, Nance DM. A randomized, double-blind, placebo-controlled, clinical study of the general effects of a standardized Lycium barbarum (Goji) Juice, GoChi. *J Altern Complement Med.* 2008 May; 14(4): 403–12.

Amagase H, Sun B, Borek C. Lycium barbarum (goji) juice improves in vivo antioxidant biomarkers in serum of healthy adults. *Nutr Res.* 2009 Jan; 29(1): 19–25.

Bucheli P, Vidal K, Shen L, Gu Z, Zhang C, Miller LE, Wang J. Goji berry effects on macular characteristics and plasma antioxidant levels. *Optom Vis Sci.* 2011 Feb; 88(2): 257–62.

Lin NC, Lin JC, Chen SH, Ho CT, Yeh AI. Effect of Goji (Lycium barbarum) on expression of genes related to cell survival. *J Agric Food Chem.* 2011 Sep 28; 59(18): 10088–96. Epub 2011 Aug 25.

Luo Q, Li Z, Yan J, Zhu F, Xu RJ, Cai YZ. Lycium barbarum polysaccharides induce apoptosis in human prostate cancer cells and inhibits prostate cancer growth in a xenograft mouse model of human prostate cancer. *J Med Food.* 2009 Aug; 12(4): 695–703.

Monzón Ballarín S, López-Matas MA, Sáenz Abad D, Pérez-Cinto N, Carnés J. Anaphylaxis associated with the ingestion of Goji berries (Lycium barbarum). *J Investig Allergol Clin Immunol.* 2011; 21(7): 567–70.

Potterat O. Goji (Lycium barbarum and L. chinense): Phytochemistry, pharmacology and safety in the perspective of traditional uses and recent popularity. *Planta Med.* 2010 Jan; 76(1): 7–19. Epub 2009 Oct 20. Review.

Reeve VE, Allanson M, Arun SJ, Domanski D, Painter N. Mice drinking goji berry juice (Lycium barbarum) are protected from UV radiation-induced skin damage via antioxidant pathways. *Photochem Photobiol Sci.* 2010 Apr; 9(4): 601–7.

Rivera CA, Ferro CL, Bursua AJ, Gerber BS. Probable Interaction Between Lycium barbarum (Goji) and Warfarin. *Pharmacotherapy.* 2012 Jan 31. doi: 10.1002/PHAR .1018. [Epub ahead of print]

Rivera CA, Ferro CL, Bursua AJ, Gerber BS. Probable interaction between Lycium barbarum (goji) and warfarin. *Pharmacotherapy.* 2012 Mar; 32(3): e50-3. doi: 10.1002/j.1875-9114.2012.01018.x.

Seeram NP. Berry fruits: compositional elements, biochemical activities, and the impact of their intake on human health, performance, and disease. *J Agric Food Chem.* 2008 Feb 13; 56(3): 627–9. Epub 2008 Jan 23.

Song MK, Roufogalis BD, Huang TH. Reversal of the Caspase-Dependent Apoptotic Cytotoxicity Pathway by Taurine from Lycium barbarum (Goji Berry) in Human Retinal Pigment Epithelial Cells: Potential Benefit in Diabetic Retinopathy. *Evid Based Complement Alternat Med.* 2012; 2012: 323784. Epub 2012 Apr 11.

Song MK, Salam NK, Roufogalis BD, Huang TH. Lycium barbarum (Goji Berry) extracts and its taurine component inhibit PPAR-γ-dependent gene transcription in human retinal pigment epithelial cells: Possible implications for diabetic retinopathy treatment. *Biochem Pharmacol.* 2011 Nov 1; 82(9): 1209–18. Epub 2011 Jul 27.

Zhang Z, Liu X, Zhang X, Liu J, Hao Y, Yang X, Wang Y. Comparative evaluation of the antioxidant effects of the natural vitamin C analog 2-O-β-D-glucopyranosyl-L-ascorbic acid isolated from Goji berry fruit. *Arch Pharm Res.* 2011 May; 34(5): 801–10. Epub 2011 Jun 9.

Goji Berries

Amagase H, Sun B, Borek C. Lycium barbarum (goji) juice improves in vivo antioxidant biomarkers in serum of healthy adults. *Nutr Res.* 2009 Jan; 29(1): 19–25.

Are some of the more exotic berry types, such as goji and açaí berries, better for health than the more common berries such as strawberries, blueberries and raspberries? *Mayo Clin Health Lett.* 2010 Nov; 28(11): 8. No abstract available.

Gómez-Bernal S, Rodríguez-Pazos L, Martínez FJ, Ginarte M, Rodríguez-Granados MT, Toribio J. Systemic photosensitivity due to Goji berries. *Photodermatol Photoimmunol Photomed.* 2011 Oct; 27(5): 245–7. doi: 10.1111/j.1600-0781.2011.00603.x.

Luo Q, Li Z, Yan J, Zhu F, Xu RJ, Cai YZ. Lycium barbarum polysaccharides induce apoptosis in human prostate cancer cells and inhibits prostate cancer growth in a xenograft mouse model of human prostate cancer. *J Med Food.* 2009 Aug; 12(4): 695–703.

Monzón Ballarín S, López-Matas MA, Sáenz Abad D, Pérez-Cinto N, Carnés J. Anaphylaxis associated with the ingestion of Goji berries (Lycium barbarum). *J Investig Allergol Clin Immunol.* 2011; 21(7): 567–70.

Navarro P, Nicolas TS, Gabaldon JA, Mercader-Ros MT, Calín-Sánchez A, Carbonell-Barrachina AA, Pérez-López AJ. Effects of cyclodextrin type on vitamin C, antioxidant activity, and sensory attributes of a mandarin juice enriched with pomegranate and goji berries. *J Food Sci.* 2011 Jun–Jul; 76(5): S319–24. doi: 10.1111/j.1750-3841.2011.02176 .x. Epub 2011 Apr 27.

Potterat O. Goji (Lycium barbarum and L. chinense): Phytochemistry, pharmacology and safety in the perspective of traditional uses and recent popularity. *Planta Med.* 2010 Jan; 76(1): 7–19. Epub 2009 Oct 20. Review.

Seeram NP. Berry fruits: compositional elements, biochemical activities, and the impact of their intake on human health, performance, and disease. *J Agric Food Chem.* 2008 Feb 13; 56(3): 627–9. Epub 2008 Jan 23.

Song MK, Roufogalis BD, Huang TH. Reversal of the Caspase-Dependent Apoptotic Cytotoxicity Pathway by Taurine from Lycium barbarum (Goji Berry) in Human Retinal Pigment Epithelial Cells: Potential Benefit in Diabetic Retinopathy. *Evid Based Complement Alternat Med.* 2012; 2012: 323784. Epub 2012 Apr 11.

Song MK, Salam NK, Roufogalis BD, Huang TH. Lycium barbarum (Goji Berry) extracts and its taurine component inhibit PPAR-γ-dependent gene transcription in human retinal pigment epithelial cells: Possible implications for diabetic retinopathy treatment. *Biochem Pharmacol.* 2011 Nov 1; 82(9): 1209–18. Epub 2011 Jul 27.

Temple NJ. The marketing of dietary supplements in North America: the emperor is (almost) naked. *J Altern Complement Med.* 2010 Jul; 16(7): 803–6.

Zhang Z, Liu X, Zhang X, Liu J, Hao Y, Yang X, Wang Y. Comparative evaluation of the antioxidant effects of the natural vitamin C analog 2-O-β-D-glucopyranosyl-L-ascorbic acid isolated from Goji berry fruit. *Arch Pharm Res.* 2011 May; 34(5): 801–10. Epub 2011 Jun 9.

Goji Berry

Amagase H, Nance DM. A randomized, double-blind, placebo-controlled, clinical study of the general effects of a standardized Lycium barbarum (Goji) Juice, GoChi. *J Altern Complement Med.* 2008 May; 14(4): 403–12.

Amagase H, Sun B, Borek C. Lycium barbarum (goji) juice improves in vivo antioxidant biomarkers in serum of healthy adults. *Nutr Res.* 2009 Jan; 29(1): 19–25.

Are some of the more exotic berry types, such as goji and açaí berries, better for health than the more common berries such as strawberries, blueberries and raspberries? *Mayo Clin Health Lett.* 2010 Nov; 28(11): 8. No abstract available.

Bucheli P, Vidal K, Shen L, Gu Z, Zhang C, Miller LE, Wang J. Goji berry effects on macular characteristics and plasma antioxidant levels. *Optom Vis Sci.* 2011 Feb; 88(2): 257–62.

Gómez-Bernal S, Rodríguez-Pazos L, Martínez FJ, Ginarte M, Rodríguez-Granados MT, Toribio J. Systemic photosensitivity due to Goji berries. *Photodermatol Photoimmunol Photomed.* 2011 Oct; 27(5): 245–7. doi: 10.1111/j.1600-0781.2011.00603.x.

J Altern Complement Med. 2010 Jul; 16(7): 803–6.

Luo Q, Li Z, Yan J, Zhu F, Xu RJ, Cai YZ. Lycium barbarum polysaccharides induce apoptosis in human prostate cancer cells and inhibits prostate cancer growth in a xenograft mouse model of human prostate cancer. *J Med Food.* 2009 Aug; 12(4): 695–703.

Monzón Ballarín S, López-Matas MA, Sáenz Abad D, Pérez-Cinto N, Carnés J. Anaphylaxis associated with the ingestion of Goji berries (Lycium barbarum). *J Investig Allergol Clin Immunol.* 2011; 21(7): 567–70.

Potterat O. Goji (Lycium barbarum and L. chinense): Phytochemistry, pharmacology and safety in the perspective of traditional uses and recent popularity. *Planta Med.* 2010 Jan; 76(1): 7–19. Epub 2009 Oct 20. Review.

Reeve VE, Allanson M, Arun SJ, Domanski D, Painter N. Mice drinking goji berry juice (Lycium barbarum) are protected from UV radiation-induced skin damage via antioxidant pathways. *Photochem Photobiol Sci.* 2010 Apr; 9(4): 601–7.

Ren Z, Na L, Xu Y, Rozati M, Wang J, Xu J, Sun C, Vidal K, Wu D, Meydani SN. Dietary Supplementation with Lacto-Wolfberry Enhances the Immune Response and Reduces Pathogenesis to Influenza Infection in Mice. *J Nutr.* 2012 Jun 27. [Epub ahead of print]

Rivera CA, Ferro CL, Bursua AJ, Gerber BS. Probable Interaction Between Lycium barbarum (Goji) and Warfarin. *Pharmacotherapy.* 2012 Jan 31. doi: 10.1002/PHAR. 1018. [Epub ahead of print]

Rivera CA, Ferro CL, Bursua AJ, Gerber BS. Probable interaction between Lycium barbarum (goji) and warfarin. *Pharmacotherapy.* 2012 Mar; 32(3): e50-3. doi: 10.1002/ j.1875-9114.2012.01018.x.

Seeram NP. Berry fruits: compositional elements, biochemical activities, and the impact of their intake on human health, performance, and disease. *J Agric Food Chem.* 2008 Feb 13; 56(3): 627–9. Epub 2008 Jan 23.

Song MK, Roufogalis BD, Huang TH. Reversal of the Caspase-Dependent Apoptotic Cytotoxicity Pathway by Taurine from Lycium barbarum (Goji Berry) in Human Retinal Pigment Epithelial Cells: Potential Benefit in Diabetic Retinopathy. *Evid Based Complement Alternat Med.* 2012; 2012: 323784. Epub 2012 Apr 11.

Song MK, Salam NK, Roufogalis BD, Huang TH. Lycium barbarum (Goji Berry) extracts and its taurine component inhibit PPAR-γ-dependent gene transcription in human retinal pigment epithelial cells: Possible implications for diabetic retinopathy treatment. *Biochem Pharmacol.* 2011 Nov 1; 82(9): 1209–18. Epub 2011 Jul 27.

Temple NJ. The marketing of dietary supplements in North America: the emperor is (almost) naked.

Zhang Z, Liu X, Zhang X, Liu J, Hao Y, Yang X, Wang Y. Comparative evaluation of the antioxidant effects of the natural vitamin C analog 2-O-β-D-glucopyranosyl-L-ascorbic acid isolated from Goji berry fruit. *Arch Pharm Res.* 2011 May; 34(5): 801–10. Epub 2011 Jun 9.

Lycium Barbarum Cancer

Cassileth B. Lycium (Lycium barbarum). *Oncology* (Williston Park). 2010 Dec; 24(14): 1353.

Chao JC, Chiang SW, Wang CC, Tsai YH, Wu MS. Hot water-extracted Lycium barbarum and Rehmannia glutinosa inhibit proliferation and induce apoptosis of hepatocellular carcinoma cells. *World J Gastroenterol.* 2006 Jul 28; 12(28): 4478–84.

Cui B, Liu S, Lin X, Wang J, Li S, Wang Q, Li S. Effects of Lycium barbarum aqueous and ethanol extracts on high-fat-diet induced oxidative stress in rat liver tissue. *Molecules.* 2011 Nov 1; 16(11): 9116-28.

Gan L, Hua Zhang S, Liang Yang X, Bi Xu H. Immunomodulation and antitumor activity by a polysaccharide-protein complex from Lycium barbarum. *Int Immunopharmacol.* 2004 Apr; 4(4): 563–9.

Gan L, Zhang SH, Liu Q, Xu HB. A polysaccharide-protein complex from Lycium barbarum upregulates cytokine expression in human peripheral blood mononuclear cells. *Eur J Pharmacol.* 2003 Jun 27; 471(3): 217–22.

Gong H, Shen P, Jin L, Xing C, Tang F. Therapeutic effects of Lycium barbarum polysaccharide (LBP) on irradiation or chemotherapy-induced myelosuppressive mice. *Cancer Biother Radiopharm.* 2005 Apr; 20(2): 155–62.

Li G, Sepkovic DW, Bradlow HL, Telang NT, Wong GY. Lycium barbarum inhibits growth of estrogen receptor positive human breast cancer cells by favorably altering estradiol metabolism. *Nutr Cancer.* 2009; 61(3): 408–14.

Luo Q, Li Z, Yan J, Zhu F, Xu RJ, Cai YZ. Lycium barbarum polysaccharides induce apoptosis in human prostate cancer cells and inhibits prostate cancer growth in a xenograft mouse model of human prostate cancer. *J Med Food.* 2009 Aug; 12(4): 695–703.

Lycium barbarum. *J Soc Integr Oncol.* 2007 Summer; 5(3): 130. No abstract available.

Mao F, Xiao B, Jiang Z, Zhao J, Huang X, Guo J. Anticancer effect of Lycium barbarum polysaccharides on colon cancer cells involves G0/G1 phase arrest. *Med Oncol.* 2011 Mar; 28(1): 121–6. Epub 2010 Jan 12.

Miao Y, Xiao B, Jiang Z, Guo Y, Mao F, Zhao J, Huang X, Guo J. Growth inhibition and cell-cycle arrest of human gastric cancer cells by Lycium barbarum polysaccharide. *Med Oncol.* 2010 Sep; 27(3): 785–90. Epub 2009 Aug 11.

Seeram NP. Berry fruits: compositional elements, biochemical activities, and the impact of their intake on human health, performance, and disease. *J Agric Food Chem.* 2008 Feb 13; 56(3): 627–9. Epub 2008 Jan 23.

Tang WM, Chan E, Kwok CY, Lee YK, Wu JH, Wan CW, Chan RY, Yu PH, Chan SW. A review of the anticancer and immunomodulatory effects of Lycium barbarum fruit. *Inflammopharmacology.* 2011 Dec 22. [Epub ahead of print]

Xin YF, Zhou GL, Deng ZY, Chen YX, Wu YG, Xu PS, Xuan YX. Protective effect of Lycium barbarum on doxorubicin-induced cardiotoxicity. *Phytother Res.* 2007 Nov; 21(11): 1020–4.

Zhang M, Chen H, Huang J, Li Z, Zhu C, Zhang S. Effect of lycium barbarum polysaccharide on human hepatoma QGY7703 cells: inhibition of proliferation and induction of apoptosis. *Life Sci.* 2005 Mar 18; 76(18): 2115–24.

Zhang Z, Liu X, Wu T, Liu J, Zhang X, Yang X, Goodheart MJ, Engelhardt JF, Wang Y. Selective suppression of cervical cancer Hela cells by 2-O-β-D-glucopyranosyl-L-ascorbic acid isolated from the fruit of Lycium barbarum L. *Cell Biol Toxicol.* 2011 Apr; 27(2): 107–21. Epub 2010 Aug 19.

Zhu CP, Zhang SH. Lycium barbarum polysaccharide inhibits the proliferation of HeLa cells by inducing apoptosis. *J Sci Food Agric.* 2012 Jun 13. doi: 10.1002/jsfa.5743. [Epub ahead of print]

INDEX

ABOUT THE AUTHOR

Dr. Earl Mindell, R.Ph., M .H., Ph.D., is generally recognized as the world's leading nutritional authority. He is the bestselling author of 55 books, including the *New Vitamin Bible*, which has sold the most books in the history of nutrition—more than 10 million copies in 34 languages, in 54 countries worldwide. His other bestsellers include *Herb Bible*, *Food as Medicine*, *Anti-Aging Bible*, *Soy Miracle*, *Allergy Bible*, *Natural Remedies for 150 Ailments* and *Prescription Alternatives*.

He has appeared on more than 1,000 radio and television programs, including *Live with Regis*, *Late Show with Letterman*, *The Oprah Winfrey Show*, *Good Morning America*, CNN and many others.

Dr. Mindell received his Bachelor of Science in Pharmacy from North Dakota State University and is currently a registered pharmacist in California. He is also a master herbalist and holds a doctorate in philosophy in nutrition.